INFORMED DECISION

THE TRUTH ABOUT CLINICAL TRIALS IN AMERICA

CALETHIA T. HODGES

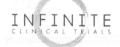

INFINITE
CLINICAL TRIALS

Published By
Infinite Clinical Trials
Morrow, GA
infiniteclinicaltrials.com

ISBN: 978-0-578-98496-4

Printed in the United States.

CONTENTS

PART I

BACKGROUND

AUTHOR'S NOTE

As a Black woman, I am no stranger to mistrust.

Being Black means operating with at least some degree of skepticism in your day-to-day life. This is, in part, an emotional and practical survival mechanism. But it is also the natural reaction to our painful history as we wait expectantly for strides that have yet to be made.

While this is not an autobiography, I'll admit that I grew up in a disadvantaged system. It was only through hard work and the grace of God that I was able to get out and make something of myself. When you grow up poor and Black, you develop a profound empathy for those in your community. You begin asking yourself hard questions. *How can I raise myself up? How can I raise my community up?*

My solution was to start a clinical trial practice. I chose this path to give back to my community and try to make things better for those in the position I once found myself. Since opening Infinite Clinical Trials, I've seen the health of individuals and our community, as a whole, changed through comprehensive, compassionate treatment.

Because of my success (and because I'm one of the few Black women in this field), I'm often interviewed and asked to speak about my insights into the clinical trials industry. During the height of the COVID-19 pandemic, the number of these interviews went up exponentially. I felt honored to have such a visible platform from which I could positively impact my community.

But since I began speaking publicly about my profession, practice, and beliefs, I have experienced a surge of negative feedback from within the Black community.

My community.

Many of the articles I was featured in communicated my desire to encourage Black individuals and communities (and minority populations in general) to participate in clinical trials. While diverse populations must be represented in clinical trials in general, it is imperative to have diversity among volunteers when developing a vaccine and treatment for a disease like COVID-19.

Almost immediately after these articles were published, I began to face backlash. Those opposed to my views accused me of everything from trying to "trick" people into being vaccinated to being a "government plant" whose goal was to harm my community. Some even assumed that by mentioning the Tuskegee "experiments" (which were not clinical trials *at all*), I was somehow commending or endorsing them. This could not be further from the truth: these experiments were nothing short of disgusting, exploitative, and morally and ethically wrong.

I was both shocked and saddened by the negativity. I couldn't believe that the mistrust in our healthcare system could extend to *me*. It truly hurt to think that I was seen as an instrument of oppression rather than an arbiter of opportunity. After all, that is what I have always tried to be.

But I realized something perhaps more eye-opening: this intense distrust of the medical research industry was, in many ways, absolutely justified. This distrust stems not only from misconceptions and misunderstandings, but also, more importantly, from a deeply rooted history of unethical and unjust treatment toward people of color. I reflected on the comments I had received and began to understand where they were coming from: systemic inequities that have been compounded and worsened by our unenviable history. When you've seen your own people treated like mere guinea pigs, it's completely understandable that willingly subjecting yourself to anything remotely similar would be out of the question.

Time and again, I've had to remind myself that most Black Americans (and Americans in general) do not have the same insights into the clinical trials industry that I do. I firmly believe that were it not for my knowledge of how clinical trials are run —my experiences with what really goes on behind closed doors —I may very well feel the same as those speaking out against me.

I soon saw that I needed to address the deep mistrust of clinical trials (and the healthcare industry as a whole) with empathy and understanding. Although this book was already in the works when I started receiving these comments, it became apparent that it wouldn't be enough to simply explain how clinical trials are run. I couldn't just broach the subject with facts, figures, and an insider's perspective. No—I needed to address and reflect on the complex set of issues that has led Black communities to fear, disdain, and denounce clinical trials for so long.

Throughout this book, I will provide my insights on what can be done to overcome the hurdles to Black participation in clinical trials—for the benefit of medical advancements and, more importantly, for the benefit of my community. As a Black, female clinician and researcher, I feel that I owe it to them to set the record straight on clinical trials and clinical research.

My goal? To encourage (not force) participation

First and foremost, participation in a clinical trial is a choice, as with any other medical treatment.

Willing participation is at the heart of clinical trials; they are entirely voluntary. For this reason, I will encourage—but never force—a person to participate in a trial. It's up to individual participants to come forward and, after learning about the specifics of a trial, decide whether to volunteer their time. Simply put, we respect everyone's individual decision to participate or not participate in clinical trials (or any form of medical treatment, for that matter). If you choose to take part in clinical trials, we will be here for you. If you choose not to, we will respect your decision completely.

As someone who has witnessed the positive impact of clinical trials firsthand, I see participation as a twofold opportunity. On the one hand, participating in a clinical trial has excellent benefits for the individual. Not only do many enrolled volunteers receive monetary compensation, but they also receive free treatments, free medication, and close clinical monitoring. In a community like mine, this can be a godsend.

Statistics show that in Atlanta, about 1 in 5 Black people is below the poverty line.[1] Furthermore, many individuals and families in my community aren't insured. I've met countless patients that require treatments and procedures they simply cannot afford to receive. Participating in clinical trials is one of the only ways that impoverished, uninsured, or otherwise disadvantaged individuals can access effective medical treatments. Not only are these treatments generally beneficial, but they're also often more effective than other available treatments. So, participants don't only get access to life-saving interventions—they also receive the most groundbreaking treatments available before they reach the rest of the population. For patients with serious medical conditions that have not yet found adequate treatment, clinical trials can significantly improve their health and overall quality of life.

On the other hand, participating in clinical trials presents individuals with an unprecedented opportunity to give back to their peers and the medical community as a whole. As I discuss throughout this book, newly developed treatments—everything from medications and surgeries to medical devices—cannot enter the market without undergoing clinical testing. Whether it's an over-the-counter allergy pill or an immunosuppressant for a chronic autoimmune disorder, every single medication you take has gone through clinical trials.

Without the participation of willing volunteers for clinical trials, new medical interventions would never be developed. Were we to find a cure for cancer, for instance, it would never reach the market without clinical trials. I say this not to guilt you into participating in a clinical trial but to show the monumental importance that participation can have in the development of life-saving treatments.

My practice is in a predominantly Black neighborhood because I want to help my community. Why do I encourage my community to participate in clinical trials? To receive free medication, free treatment, compensation, and to help the community as a whole. Ultimately, however, participation in a clinical trial is your choice.

On the Tuskegee syphilis experiments

In one interview with NBC,[2] I referenced a series of experiments conducted over the course of several decades, from the 1930s to the 1970s. These experiments—the Tuskegee syphilis experiments, often incorrectly referred to as "clinical trials"—promised treatment for "bad blood," an umbrella term to refer to a number of diseases, including syphilis.[3]

Working with the Tuskegee Institute, a historically Black university in Tuskegee, Alabama, the United States Public Health Service recruited 600 Black men to participate in the trials. They agreed, of course, only under the assumption that they would receive beneficial treatments. In a show of complete disregard for clinical integrity, researchers never gave the men adequate treatment for syphilis. Even after penicillin became the first line of treatment for the disease, these participants never received it. In fact, the study's advisory panel found no evidence that the men were given a choice to quit the study either before or after penicillin was established as an effective treatment for syphilis.

I used the Tuskegee "clinical trials" in my interview as an example of why Black Americans have every right to mistrust the clinical research industry. These "clinical trials" were, at their core, exploitative experiments on unwilling participants. These men were treated like lab rats, unknowingly participating in malicious studies they were told were for their own good for over 40 years.

I am disgusted by the Tuskegee experiments—and by many other examples throughout history—because of the unethical, blatant disregard for human rights that have occurred in clinical research.

So, how are real clinical trials different? All participants in a real clinical trial receive informed consent. In short, they must be made completely aware of what they are agreeing to participate in, including all of the risks and benefits of the treatments being administered. No patient can ever participate in a clinical trial without fully understanding what will go on during the trial and what treatments they are going to receive.

In the case of the Tuskegee experiments, no evidence was found that the researchers conducting the experiments had informed the participants of the study or its true purpose. In fact, the men participating weren't even given enough information to provide informed consent and were actually lied to by the researchers.

Ultimately, an out-of-court settlement worth $10 million was filed in an attempt to make reparations for the wrongs that had been done to these men and their families. But in my opinion, money—no matter how much—will never be enough to repair such deeply damaged trust.

While I cannot know what it was like to be so intentionally taken advantage of, I empathize with the pain these men and their families experienced. I believe that it's up to people like me

—and anyone who understands the long, complicated, and often painful history of being Black in America—to right these wrongs from the inside out.

My purpose in writing this book

I opened my practice, in part, because I want to help rebuild this broken trust through compassionate, transparent care. I know that members of the Black community are tired of being told to trust the healthcare industry by those who could not even begin to understand the pain and mistrust they feel.

As a Black American myself, I aim to foster a sense of trust, community, and understanding with my patients. But while this is a personal goal for my practice, I feel that I can do more to begin dispelling the myths and righting the wrongs that have followed the clinical trials industry for so long. As someone who belongs to both the Black community and the medical community, I feel a sense of personal responsibility to heal the rift between them.

I hope that, as a Black woman, members of the Black community will consider what I have to say with open minds. I hope that, as the owner of a clinical trials practice, readers will trust that my knowledge and experience inform everything I've written here. And I hope, above all, to leave you better informed and more prepared when deciding whether to participate in clinical trials.

INTRODUCTION

It would be hard to overstate how pleased I am that this book has finally seen the light of day. Between running my clinical trial practice, Infinite Clinical Trials, and managing a family, it's been a long time coming.

Granted, there's no shortage of research, discussion, and writing on the subject of clinical trials. Throughout all my years in healthcare, however, I've noticed a trend: the majority of the literature on clinical trials is not intended for the general public. Much of the literature is clinician-facing (e.g., how to start your own clinical trial or the best legal and ethical practices for conducting clinical trials). These topics, while helpful for researchers and clinicians, are mostly irrelevant to the generic public. This type of writing tends to be too dry, academic, and inaccessible to most people who might benefit from participation in clinical trials.

My goal is to present clinical trials in a way that everyone can understand and benefit from. Just as it's my professional responsibility to ensure that new treatments help improve the health of individuals and populations, I believe that it's my personal responsibility to shed light on the truth about clinical trials. With this book, I hope to spread awareness—and a better understanding—of the importance of clinical trials.

I also hope to debunk some of the myths surrounding clinical trials. Unfortunately, many people believe that participating in a clinical trial is like volunteering to be a lab rat or guinea pig. They believe that the treatments being tested are unsafe or won't work, that you have to be terminally ill in order to participate in a clinical trial, or that participants won't be able to continue receiving treatment—even if it proves successful—once the trial has ended. Thankfully, none of this is true.

Most of all, I hope to help improve participation in clinical trials—especially among minorities. As a woman of color, the lack of diverse representation among participants in clinical trials hits especially close to home. I hope to see more representation —not only because minority populations have unique reactions to certain treatments (making their active participation in clinical trials so crucial), but also because diversity within medical studies is necessary to develop new treatments that benefit as much of the population as possible. For the sake of safety, public health, and equal representation, it's my goal to contribute to increased clinical trial participation within communities of color.

Finally, if you enjoy this book, I highly recommend that you read *The Gift of Participation* by Ken Getz. I can't recommend it enough. One of the biggest struggles I have faced is getting people outside of my field to understand the huge importance of clinical trials. There's so much stigma and fear, which is a shame, as clinical trials save lives. Getz's book helps to alleviate much of that negativity. It showcases how clinical trials can have a profound impact on health outcomes—not just in participants, but in people across the world.

WHAT ARE CLINICAL TRIALS?

There are two main types of clinical studies: observational studies and interventional studies.

As their name suggests, observational studies are all about *observation* (rather than intervention or treatment). There are many reasons why investigators may choose to hold observational studies.

Say, for example, investigators wanted to determine the health effects of the legalization of cannabis on a particular community. Conducting a conventional randomized experiment to do so would be difficult for multiple reasons. For one, the investigators most likely don't have the power to enact this law across numerous communities. Additionally, the ethics of assigning one randomly chosen group of subjects to consume cannabis (while the other abstains from it) would be questionable. Instead, the investigators would choose to observe and record the health effects of legalizing cannabis within a community that has already done so. So, rather than intervening (by prescribing changes in treatments, environment, or other similar factors), investigators in observational studies simply "let nature run its course" and observe the results of these changes on the participants.

What we're discussing in this book, however, are interventional studies—more commonly known as clinical trials.

In short, a clinical trial is a series of tests of a newly developed treatment conducted on human participants. This treatment may take any form, from a medication to a surgical procedure, or even a behavioral intervention (like a new exercise regimen). Unlike observational studies, clinical trials involve *intervening* with a participant's course of treatment—by administering a new procedure, drug, medical device, or activity—and observing the results. These results are used to determine whether a potential treatment will be approved for use by the general public.

There are two key reasons why clinical trials are held. The first is that new medical treatments can't reach the market until they've undergone testing in clinical trials. If it weren't for clinical testing, medical professionals wouldn't be able to determine whether a potential treatment is safe, effective, and practical enough for public use. That's why passing clinical trials is such a major hurdle—one that must be cleared before a treatment is approved for the market. Without clinical trials, many advances in medicine would never see the light of day.

The second factor that makes clinical trials so important is that they help the medical community make strides in providing more effective treatments. Clinical trials are necessary in order to develop new treatments for all forms of diseases, from congenital conditions present at birth to aggressive forms of cancer. Not only is this essential to maintaining a healthy population, but it's also vital to improving quality of life for people living with debilitating diseases. Some clinical trials are conducted not to directly benefit participants but with the intention of helping scientists and medical professionals come up with better, more effective treatments for future patients.

Clinical research

A clinical trial is just one aspect of a larger process known as *clinical research.* This process is used to develop the treatments that will be tested in clinical trials. By definition, clinical research refers to all types of research carried out on human participants. The main goal of clinical research is to increase the medical community's understanding of specific diseases and conditions and to improve treatment approaches.

There are many different forms of clinical research. Genetic studies, for example, aim to identify the link between genetics and certain health conditions. This is done in the hopes of improving prediction and early detection. Treatment research and prevention research, on the other hand, seek to improve medical interventions and preventative measures that stop diseases from developing or recurring. These forms of research may incorporate a wide variety of treatments—including radiation therapy, medication, vitamins and minerals, psychotherapy, and lifestyle changes (such as diet changes or smoking cessation) —to improve the lives of people living with specific conditions or diseases.

Ultimately, clinical trials can be thought of as practical, real-world applications of clinical research. That's why they're also known as *clinical research studies.* After researchers devise new procedures or experimental treatments, they proceed to testing through clinical trials. During the testing process, critical information regarding efficacy, safety, and practicality—as well as the viability of other potential treatments—is obtained.

The phases of clinical trials

Clinical trials only begin after a period of *preclinical research* is conducted. Unlike clinical trials, preclinical research is not performed with human participants. Instead, it analyzes different aspects of a newly developed treatment, such as the components of its chemical makeup or how it interacts with the human body. After the preclinical research phase has been completed, the experimental treatment moves on to a series of clinical trials.

The United States Food and Drug Administration (FDA) has defined[1] what are commonly considered the five phases of clinical trials. Multiple trials are held during each of these phases:

- **Phase 0 trials:** An exploratory study of the experimental drug or treatment is conducted with very limited human exposure to the drug. No therapeutic or diagnostic goals are set during this stage.
- **Phase I trials:** The experimental drug or treatment is tested for the first time on a small group of participants. During this phase, researchers test the safety of the treatment, determine the drug's safe dosage range (if the trial involves medication), and identify any side effects.
- **Phase II trials:** The experimental treatment is administered to a larger group of people with the aim of determining whether it's effective and to further evaluate its safety. Some Phase II trials are further divided into Phase IIA, during which researchers assess how much of a drug should be administered, and Phase IIB, when they assess how well a drug works at the prescribed dosage.
- **Phase III trials:** The experimental treatment is administered to several larger groups of participants. At this stage, researchers confirm how effective the drug is, compare its safety and efficacy to available treatments, monitor any side effects that occur, and collect vital information that will allow the

experimental treatment to be used safely on an even larger population.

- **Phase IV trials:** The final trial phase involves conducting studies on very large groups (up to thousands of patients) after the treatment has been approved for general use by the FDA. These studies, called "post-marketing studies," help provide further information about the treatment, including its risks, benefits, and best use cases.

This is the typical progression of clinical trials for newly developed medications and drug treatments. The process may look a little different for other experimental interventions, such as medical devices.

Each phase of a clinical trial builds on the ones that came before it and is designed to answer specific questions about the treatment being tested. The pros and cons of participating in each phase will be discussed in detail during the trial's informed consent process.

How are clinical trials conducted?

When we discuss the myths and misconceptions surrounding clinical trials later in this book, you'll see what it's actually like to participate in a clinical trial. For now, let's briefly review how clinical trials are run.

First and foremost, clinical trials are performed only on willing participants. This means that each individual taking part in a trial has volunteered to participate. When participating in a clinical trial, volunteers agree to receive one or more treatments (interventions) or a placebo. A placebo is a "fake" treatment given to one group of participants (called the control group). In other words, the control group is not receiving any treatment and instead serves as the "base case" against which the group receiving the real treatment is compared.

Clinical trials can be conducted in many different locations. Commonly, they take place in hospitals, universities, community clinics, and third-party clinical testing labs (like Infinite Clinical Trials). A clinical trial may also be *inpatient,* meaning participants stay overnight in the research center or hospital, or *outpatient,* meaning participants can return home at the end of the day. Additionally, there's no set time frame for clinical trials— your participation in the trial may take anywhere from a few weeks to several years. That's why, when researching a clinical trial, it's very important that you take all these different factors into consideration before deciding whether to participate.

Informed consent

Clinical trial participants are made aware of much of a trial's protocol, or set research plan, before getting started. This protocol, which is designed to answer particular research questions (as well as protect the health and wellness of participants), usually addresses the following[2]:

- The purpose of the trial
- The length of the trial
- Who may participate in the trial (called the *eligibility criteria*—more on this later)
- The number of participants needed for the trial
- What information is gathered from participants
- The schedule of procedures, tests, or drugs and each of their dosages

If you were to participate in a clinical trial, you probably wouldn't hear the word "protocol" in discussions with clinicians or researchers. That's because, when talking to participants, we usually use the term "informed consent" instead. Informed consent refers to both the process of obtaining consent from clinical trial participants as well as the physical document they must sign in order to participate.

An informed consent form, or ICF, includes all the information you need before making this decision. It outlines all known information about the safety, viability, and potential effectiveness of the experimental treatment in question. It also describes the purpose of the clinical trial, the exact number of visits that are required, the types of procedures that will be performed, and the timeline during which the trial will take place. Finally, the ICF explains all the possible risks and benefits of participating in the trial.

Some people worry that by signing an ICF, they're signing their rights away on something they don't fully understand. Luckily, these documents are always written in layperson terms so they can be easily understood by participants without a scientific or medical background. This ensures that participants are truly offered informed consent—that they agree to participate in good faith and with a full understanding of what they are signing up for.

Informed consent involves much more than just reading and signing a document. The second key component of informed consent is the process of informed consent. This process is the ongoing explanation of all aspects of a clinical trial. We say "ongoing" because informed consent never really stops at any one point during the trial. Even after researchers have provided participants with all the information they have, there is a continuous effort to make sure that trial participants know their rights, understand the potential benefits and risks of the treatment, and have all their questions answered in a timely manner.

The goal of the informed consent process is to ensure that participants understand every aspect of a clinical trial—before, during, and after making the decision to participate. As the FDA states, informed consent is not just providing a one-time information session or signing a single document, but engaging in an ongoing, interactive discussion.[3] By providing continuous information on the trial, researchers help participants make the most well-informed decisions on whether they'd like to begin—or continue—participating.

Confidentiality, rules, and guidelines

Clinical trials are often sponsored by a wide variety of institutions. Pharmaceutical firms, federal agencies (such as the National Institutes of Health), academic or independent medical centers, volunteer groups, and even private individuals or companies may all lend funding and support to a clinical trial.

Additionally, the specific details of how a particular clinical trial is run (such as whether it's conducted in an inpatient or outpatient setting) can vary. Regardless, strict rules have been put in place to govern how all clinical research and trials are conducted. These rules, established by the FDA and National Institutes of Health (NIH), help ensure that clinical trials follow rigorous standards of safety and ethics.

One of the main components of these standards in clinical trials is Good Clinical Practice (GCP). According to the FDA, GCP is defined as[4] "a standard for the design, conduct, performance, monitoring, auditing, recording, analysis and reporting of clinical trials and studies." In other words, GCP is a quality standard that helps ensure that the rights, safety, and well-being of all participants in clinical trials are protected. Clinical trial practices take GCP very seriously. At my practice, for instance, the investigators and clinical research staff responsible for managing and conducting trials aren't just trained once in GCP. They receive ongoing training and undergo annual testing for annual recertification.

As with any medical procedure or practice, confidentiality is crucial when it comes to clinical trials. The personal and medical information of all participants in clinical trials is kept confidential throughout the entire process and is only available to researchers and patients themselves. When the results of clinical trials are published, they are usually presented as overall conclusions without referring to individual participants.

According to the 2003 Health Insurance Portability and Accountability Act (HIPAA) Privacy Rule, informed consent involves more than just maintaining the confidentiality of participant health records—all identifying medical information of participants must be kept confidential.[5] This information, referred to as "protected health information," exceeds a patient's medical records to include any identifying information (there are a total of 18 identifiers, including participant name and medical record number).

Informed consent regulations mandate that all ICFs contain statements outlining the specific extent to which identifying records will be kept confidential. Most ICFs also include an "authorization" (namely, HIPAA Authorization to Use and Disclose Protected Health Information).[6] An authorization is a detailed document that provides the people running a clinical trial permission to use a participant's protected health information for specific purposes. An authorization will answer questions such as:

- What particular information can be used and disclosed?
- Who is authorized to do so?
- For how long?
- For what purpose will the information be used and disclosed?

Additionally, authorizations should also explain the participant's right to revoke their authorization at any time and describe how they can go about doing so. Volunteers should have all their questions answered and be completely informed about their rights, privacy, and participation before, during, and after a clinical trial.

THE HISTORY OF CLINICAL TRIALS

Now that we have a baseline understanding of what clinical trials are and how they work, let's take a look at their history. From the first recorded trials in biblical times to modern-day clinical trials, the scientific, ethical, and regulatory practices surrounding clinical trials have changed dramatically over time.

While the focus of this book isn't on the evolution of medical practices or the scientific method, touching upon the origins and development of clinical trials will give us a better understanding of how they work today. (And the next time it's International Clinical Trials Day [May 20th], you'll know exactly what achievements we're celebrating.)

Clinical trials in ancient history

The *first-ever* documented experiment that resembled a clinical trial was recorded in the Book of Daniel in the Bible.[1] This experiment, conducted by King Nebuchadnezzar, took place in Babylon around 500 BCE. According to records, Nebuchadnezzar, in an effort to keep his people in peak physical condition, ordered them to consume a diet of only meat and wine. After some protested eating meat, the king allowed certain individuals to follow a diet consisting of legumes and water on one condition: he would assess their health after ten days. At the end of this "trial period," those who consumed the alternative diet appeared to be better nourished than their meat-eating, wine-drinking peers. Despite his dismay, Nebuchadnezzar changed his public health policy, permitting the vegetarian diet and ordering a reduction in the consumption of wine. This experiment, while rudimentary, may very well have been one of the first times in which a human experiment was used to guide decisions about public health.

More than a millennium later, in 1025 AD, the hugely influential Persian philosopher Avicenna wrote on the testing of health treatments. In his *Canon of Medicine* (which was used as the standard medical textbook in both Islamic and Christian countries until the 18th century), Avicenna suggested that when studying a drug, two opposing cases should be observed, as well as the time of action and reproducibility of the drug's effects. While there seems to be no record of the practical application of these rules, they are surprisingly similar to the modern approaches taken to conduct clinical trials.

These early examples of interventional studies lack many of the features of modern and much more rigorous clinical trials. Ancient medical investigations were largely based on trial and error, observation, and anecdotal evidence—the Babylonians, for example, were reported to exhibit ailing citizens in public spaces so that passersby could offer medical advice based on their personal experiences with similar illnesses.[2] All that aside, writings like Avicenna's and "clinical trials" like Nebuchadnezzar's set the stage for the modern methods and applications of clinical trials today.

Origins, development, and the first controlled trial: 16th–18th centuries

As medical knowledge advanced and medical practices grew more sophisticated, trying out new interventions on a smaller test group became increasingly common. As we'll see, however, the majority of these early experiments lacked the checks and balances we use today to ensure that the results of clinical trials are reliable. These pseudo-clinical trials were not randomized, controlled, or blinded.

The first-ever clinical trial of a newly developed medical intervention is typically attributed to Ambroise Paré, the official surgeon to the kings of France.[3] In 1537, Paré was serving as a military surgeon, helping treat soldiers wounded in battle. At this time, the customary practice to prevent battle wounds from getting infected was to douse them with boiling oil. One day, as the number of casualties mounted, Paré found that the oil had run out. In its place, he prepared and administered an ancient Roman treatment consisting of egg yolk, turpentine, and the oil of roses.

Paré rose early the next morning to check up on the soldiers who had received this new treatment, worried that it would not prove as effective as boiling oil. Much to his surprise, the new treatment appeared more effective than the customary one. Paré found that the soldiers who had received the boiling oil were "feverish with much pain and swelling about their wounds," while those to whom he applied the Roman mixture were "feeling but little pain, their wounds neither swollen nor inflamed." At that moment, Paré determined that he would never again "burn thus so cruelly the poor wounded" with the oil treatment.

One particularly noteworthy prelude to modern clinical trials was conducted nearly 200 years later by British author Lady Mary Wortley Montagu (1689–1762)[4]. Lady Mary, whose complexion had been marred by a severe case of smallpox in her youth,[5] championed the inoculation (then called variolation) against smallpox in England. Having observed the practice during a visit to Turkey, she hoped to help prevent the ravages of the disease in her home country. After having her five-year-old son and four-year-old daughter successfully inoculated with the disease (in 1718 and 1721)[6], Lady Mary campaigned for further study of variolation.

Thanks to her advocacy, many such experiments proceeded. One experiment, which occurred after word of the practice had reached the royal family, involved a unique arrangement. Several prisoners sentenced to execution agreed to undergo variolation in exchange for the king's pardon from death row. After receiving the inoculation, all of the prisoners survived, and those who were later exposed to smallpox proved to be immune to the disease. Similar effective experiments were performed by Edward Jenner, who, as an eight-year-old boy in 1757, was one of the thousands of English children to be inoculated with smallpox.

Despite these success stories, none of these experiments definitively proved that inoculation was effective at preventing smallpox. Because no control group was used, there was no way to assess whether immunity resulted from variolation or from other unidentified factors. While it may seem like common sense to assume that it was Paré's new treatment that soothed his soldiers' wounds or variolation that protected recipients from smallpox, such experiments wouldn't hold up today. They lack the safeguards needed to *accurately* demonstrate the effectiveness of the interventions being tested: randomization, blinding, and control groups.

James Lind and scurvy: the first controlled clinical trial in history

The first proper clinical trial (that had most of the elements of a controlled trial) took place in 1747[7]. This famous trial, conducted by British naval surgeon James Lind, was a bit unconventional: it took place not in a carefully monitored lab or medical environment but on a ship at sea.

At the time, scurvy—a disease now known to be caused by vitamin C deficiency—was a common affliction among sailors on long-distance ocean voyages. Just seven years prior to Lind's experiment, the disease had wreaked havoc on a fleet of British ships circumnavigating the globe. Of the 1,900 men aboard Commodore George Anson's eight ships, 1,400 (nearly three-quarters) had died, the majority allegedly from scurvy.[8]

Lind was mortified. Hoping to prevent the same fate among his crew aboard the *HMS Salisbury*, Lind planned a trial to compare the effectiveness of several popular contemporary remedies for scurvy. He selected 12 men, all suffering from similar symptoms of scurvy (which, according to his original notes, included "putrid gums, the spots and lassitude, with weakness of the knees"[9]). He divided these men into six pairs, each of which received one of the following suggested treatments:

- One quart of cider per day
- One half-pint of seawater per day
- 25 drops of elixir of vitriol (sulfuric acid and alcohol) 3 times per day
- Two spoonfuls of vinegar 3 times per day
- A "nutmeg-sized" paste of mustard seed, horseradish, garlic, and tree sap 3 times per day
- Two oranges and one lemon per day

We know today that the last treatment—thanks to the high vitamin C content in citrus fruits—proved most effective in combating scurvy. However, while fellow British military surgeon John Woodall had already recommended eating citrus fruits to prevent scurvy as early as the 17th century, the practice didn't catch on.[10] But Lind's results were clear: after six days, one of the two men who had consumed the oranges and lemons had recovered enough to care for the rest of the sick, while the other had made a complete recovery. Thanks to Lind's findings, the British navy started supplying citrus to its ships in 1795.[11]

Aside from his findings, what was so important about Lind's trial was that it was controlled. His trial was an example of a "parallel-arm experiment" (one in which participants are divided into two or more groups). In fact, it was the first of its kind. In an ideal world, the members of each of the groups participating in a parallel-arm experiment would be identical in every way. While it's not realistically possible to achieve this, Lind was careful to ensure that variations in external factors wouldn't interfere with his results (that's why he had two men assigned to each diet in question). By maintaining this consistency across the study, James Lind performed the first recorded, controlled clinical trial in history.

Modern clinical trials take shape: 19th century to present day

The foundations of modern clinical trials had already started to form by the time of Lind's trial in the 18th century. More than 100 years later, in the 1860s, British physician Sir William Gull continued the work begun by John Haygarth on a fraudulent medical device (the Perkin's Patent Tractors), demonstrating the importance of control groups to correctly identifying the placebo effect.[11] In the same century, Frederick Akbar Mahomed (of Guy's Hospital, London) performed detailed clinical trials on high blood pressure and founded the Collective Investigation Record for the British Medical Association, which served as the foundation of today's collaborative clinical trials.[12]

As reported by medical historian Harry Marks, it was in post-WWII America that statistics-driven randomized clinical trials (RCTs) came to the forefront of evidence-based medicine.[18] Even before then, interest in clinical research and trials had started to grow, in part, thanks to the huge medical and scientific advances that had been made (including the discovery of microbes and the development of vaccines for rabies and anthrax). But interest wasn't the only motivation—Americans desperately needed quality clinical trials. At the time, medical treatments in the United States were more or less a sham: at the turn of the 19th century, the sale of "patent medicines" (a misnomer if there ever was one, as only the bottle and label containing these drugs were patented or trademarked) made up 72% of all drug sales in the country.

In 1920s Britain, statistician Sir Ronald A. Fisher developed his *Principles of Experimental Design*, a work outlining the best practices for designing experiments. His principles included many of those at the forefront of today's clinical trials, such as randomization (the random assignment of participants to different experimental groups) and replication (the repetition and replication of measurements and experiments in order to identify areas of variation, reducing uncertainty in the results). These principles were further explored by fellow statistician Sir Austin Bradford Hill, who reached widespread renown thanks to his landmark study in the 1950s with Richard Doll on the correlation between smoking and lung cancer.

Streptomycin and the first randomized controlled trial

As researchers further improved their methods, clinical trials became increasingly more accurate, sophisticated, and influential. It was the first randomized controlled trial on streptomycin, however, that has remained one of the most groundbreaking trials in history.[13]

Following the monumental discovery of penicillin by Alexander Fleming in 1928, a great deal of research was conducted to identify other potential antibiotics that might be effective in treating bacterial infections. One of these infections was pulmonary tuberculosis, which penicillin was unable to treat. Tuberculosis was, at the time, the "most important" cause of death among young adults in North America and Europe (and, according to the World Health Organization, still remains the leading cause of death from a single infectious agent[14]).

From 1946–47, English pulmonologist Sir Geoffrey Marshall carried out a clinical trial to test whether a newly developed antibiotic, streptomycin, would be effective in curing pulmonary tuberculosis. There were two key elements that allowed this trial to be considered the first randomized curative trial.[15] Firstly, it was placebo-controlled. This meant that one group of patients received the experimental treatment (streptomycin), while another received a placebo—a harmless pill that would not have any effects on the patients. The placebo group served as a control, and their results could be compared to those of the group receiving streptomycin. Secondly, the experiment was double-blind: neither the participants nor the doctors monitoring them knew which patients received streptomycin and which received a placebo.

An advisory committee formed for Marshall's trial decided that a series of multi-center trials would be carried out at several tuberculosis units throughout the U.K. It was determined that both groups of participants would receive the current standard treatment for pulmonary tuberculosis (bed rest) while just one would receive the experimental antibiotic. As is the case with clinical trials today, Marshall's trial included a set of eligibility criteria:

- When a consultant physician determined that a patient was potentially eligible for the trial, the patient's details were forwarded to the trial's national coordinating center.
- If they were found to meet the trial's eligibility criteria, they were arranged to be admitted to the next available hospital bed in the nearest participating center. (Due to a limited supply of hospital beds, the patients receiving bed rest alone were given priority admission.)

- If streptomycin was found to be effective in the other group of patients, those on bed rest would receive it in the future when a larger supply of the drug became available.

At the participating trial centers, each gender was allotted a set of randomly numbered envelopes containing cards indicating "S" (streptomycin) or "C" (control). While streptomycin and control patients were generally admitted to different wards, they were treated exactly the same so as to ensure consistency and accuracy in the trial's results. Throughout the trial, patient progress was assessed with monthly chest X-rays, evaluated by three specialists who remained blind to (unaware of) which patients had been given streptomycin and bed rest and which patients had been given bed rest alone. Cultures of patient sputum (saliva and mucus) were similarly evaluated by bacteriologists blinded to the patients' treatments.

The trial ultimately proved the efficacy of streptomycin in treating pulmonary tuberculosis and improving patient health outcomes. In the six months following the trial, 4 deaths occurred among the 55 patients who had received streptomycin (7.27%), compared to 15 deaths among the 52 patients who received bed rest alone (27.27%). But the study revealed much more than just a new treatment for tuberculosis: it also uncovered vital information about the development of resistance to streptomycin.

Antibiotic resistance occurs when bacteria evolve ways of protecting themselves against the drugs administered to kill them. At the time of Marshall's trial, the development of antibiotic resistance in individual patients was a new phenomenon—it had not occurred in individuals who had taken penicillin. After researchers witnessed this antibiotic resistance, it was determined that physicians could not rely on streptomycin alone to cure tuberculosis. It was soon found that combining streptomycin with another new drug, para-aminosalicylic acid (PAS), was much more effective in treating tuberculosis than either medication alone. Using this combination of drugs also reduced the development of antibiotic resistance.

Marshall's trial proved invaluable in advancing our understanding of drug-resistant illnesses. Perhaps more importantly, the results of randomized trials like this Marshall's, coupled with further research into drug resistance, allowed his research team to achieve 100% cure rates for pulmonary tuberculosis—the most common form of a disease which, until then, had killed half of all people who caught it.

The streptomycin trial was groundbreaking and set the stage for clinical trials for years to come. As John Crofton, one of the researchers leading the trial, wrote, "For many of those of us who had been involved in the MRC streptomycin trial, randomized trials became a way of life, and provided much of the evidence upon which rational treatment policies came to be based."

The Tuskegee syphilis experiments and beyond: exploitation and mistrust in American medical research

The Tuskegee Syphilis Study—often misidentified as a clinical trial—remains at the forefront of Black Americans' consciousnesses to this day. While I explained the study in more detail in my Author's Note, the bottom line is that the study's researchers knowingly denied unwitting Black men with syphilis the lifesaving treatments they needed. The exploitative study was not in any way a clinical trial and was absolutely the exception—not the rule—to the way in which proper, ethical clinical trials are conducted in America.

But despite the improvements that have been made in ensuring ethical, consensual clinical trials, we cannot discount the deep, lasting impacts experiments like these have on subjects, their families, and Black Americans as a whole. The effect this experimentation has had on Black American perceptions of the healthcare and medical research industries has been heartbreaking. The Tuskegee experiments contributed to one of the most common fears among people of color: volunteering for clinical trials is akin to signing their rights away and allowing predatory researchers to profit off treating them like "lab rats" or "guinea pigs." Knowing that Black people have been taken advantage of like this is bad enough. But to voluntarily put themselves through what they see as an exploitative process—to trust the system that betrayed them—would be foolish. This opinion is most evident in the disproportionate lack of representation of people of color within clinical studies—especially when some studies could benefit them the most.

Consider the clinical trials for Ninlaro—a drug approved by the FDA in 2015 for the serious blood cancer multiple myeloma. While Black Americans are more than two times more likely to be diagnosed with this cancer than their White peers, only 13 of the trial's 722 participants (1.8%) were Black. Furthermore, analysis of FDA data found that in 24 of the 31 clinical trials for cancer drugs approved between 2015–2018, fewer than 5% of participants were Black.[16]

But to write this lack of participation off as Black Americans simply failing to take advantage of "great opportunities" would be a gross oversimplification of many complex, multilayered issues. The so-called "misconceptions" about clinical trials that prevail among many people of color are not merely based on a lack of understanding—in many cases, they stem from deeply rooted (and entirely justified) mistrust. This mistrust extends far beyond the painful memory of the Tuskegee experiments. Some causes of this mistrust are easier to identify than others.

As we see in *More Than Tuskegee: Understanding Mistrust About Research Participation* (D.P. Scharff, Ph.D. et al.), more than 400 years of government-sanctioned exploitation has left Black Americans unwilling to contribute to clinical research. Time and time again, their participation has left them worse for wear. As recently as the 1990s, for example, a study on aggressive behavior among African American boys offered parents significant monetary incentives to enroll their children in a trial. After enrollment, these boys were subjected to significant human rights violations, such as the withholding of water and withdrawal of crucial medications the boys were taking, including asthma medications.

A myriad of complex issues and causes have deepened the rift between Black Americans and the medical industry. Despite making strides to provide equity in other areas of life, disparities between health and access to healthcare still exist between different races and social classes to this day. In particular, patients of ethnic minority backgrounds have been found to receive less comprehensive information, attention, and empathy from their physicians than their White counterparts.[17,18]

Additionally, many people in minority communities do not trust the federal government. Some feel that the government has failed them, taken advantage of them, and oppressed them. Some look at deplorable occurrences like the Tuskegee experiments and have no desire to further the aims of an institution capable of such actions. And because minority communities often associate medical research with the same government that has lost their trust—or has failed to earn their trust in the first place—they see no reason to trust medical researchers, either.

Black people are also aware that some clinical research is inherently biased in the way it's set up. For instance, many clinical trials include eligibility criteria for age. Let's say the minimum age requirement for a trial on a new hypertension (high blood pressure) treatment for American adults is 50 years old. Because Black people tend to have an earlier onset of hypertension than White people, such biased criteria would prevent many Black Americans who could benefit from participating.[19] By the time they've reached 50 years of age, many Black Americans may be ineligible for such a trial because their disease has become too severe for them to participate.

Even when Black people do participate in studies, these

studies may not consider the ways that people of color see the world or perform everyday tasks. As cited in *More Than Tuskegee*, for instance, a Black man was interested in participating in a study about razor burn but was dismayed to find that researchers were not familiar with hair-removal techniques common in the Black community.

When a study appears to be designed to keep certain participants out, people will start to wonder whether clinical research has their best interests at heart. Unfortunately, history has given many African Americans plenty of reasons not to participate in clinical trials, which is why they continue to participate at lower rates than White Americans.

Ethical advancements

It was in direct response to exploitative medical experimentation like the Tuskegee syphilis experiments that legislation has been passed to protect individual rights and ensure more ethical clinical trials. In 1974, two years after the Tuskegee experiments ended, the United States Congress signed the National Research Act into law, creating the National Commission for the Protection of Human Subjects of Biomedical and Behavioral Research.[20] This commission's purpose was to identify the basic principles regarding ethics and patient rights that would govern all future medical and behavioral studies on human subjects. It developed guidelines for how to properly select participants for clinical trials and defined how informed consent should be provided and obtained in different research settings. The commission also had the responsibility of developing guidelines to ensure that all members of the medical community adhere to the principles set forth.

While the commission helped devise guidelines for informed consent in clinical trials, regulations were also passed in 1974 requiring researchers to obtain voluntary informed consent from all participants in clinical trials performed or funded by the

United States Department of Health, Education, and Welfare (DHEW). These regulations require that all DHEW-supported studies on human participants undergo review by institutional review boards (IRBs), which are responsible for reviewing clinical trial protocols and determining whether they meet ethical standards. Today, the Department of Health and Human Services Office for Human Research Protections oversees all aspects of clinical trials, including informed consent, communication of diagnosis, and accurate reporting of test results.

Efforts to maintain ethical clinical trials are still ongoing. Since the enactment of the National Research Act, the rules and regulations surrounding human research have been reviewed and revised to reflect our refined understanding of ethical patient protections. In the late 1970s, for instance, an ethics advisory board was formed to further review ethics in biomedical research. From 1980–83, the President's Commission for the Study of Ethical Problems in Medicine and Biomedical and Behavioral Research evaluated how closely researchers were adhering to federal rules for studies involving human participants. In 1991, a total of 16 federal departments and agencies adopted the Federal Policy for the Protection of Human Subjects (also known as the "Common Rule"). In 1995, a National Bioethics Advisory Commission was formed to ensure that current regulations, policies, and procedures had all possible safeguards in place to protect research participants. This commission was succeeded by the President's Council on Bioethics in 2001 and the Presidential Commission for the Study of Bioethical Issues in 2009.

Each of these commissions, review boards, and acts aims to uphold "good clinical practice" (GCP). In short, good clinical practice is the principle governing everything we do in clinical research. At Infinite Clinical Trials, for instance, my staff must keep an updated certificate attesting to our adherence to GCP. This certificate must be renewed every two years. Following good clinical practice is just one of many ways to ensure that we take the utmost care to protect the rights of patients, keep their information secure and confidential, and ensure that all clinical trials are conducted properly and ethically. It is my responsibility and duty to do so—not just as a member of the Association of Clinical Research Professionals, but as a woman who has vowed to treat each and every patient with the respect, integrity, and compassion they deserve.

WHY ARE CLINICAL TRIALS IMPORTANT?

Think about a medication you or a loved one have taken recently. This could be a prescription (such as antibiotics for an infection), an over-the-counter medication (like pain relievers), or even a dietary supplement. Chances are, you glanced over the label. If you've ever taken a closer look at the labels on your medications and supplements, however, you've probably noticed something: they're all pretty much the same.

Over-the-counter medication labels generally include a product's "drug facts"—active ingredient[s], amounts, purposes—as well as uses, directions, warnings, and additional information. Prescription treatments may include important warning information (such as "take with food" or "for oral use only") alongside the medication's generic and brand names, dosage, and dosing schedule. You may have also noticed that certain dietary supplements include similar labels. Some have a disclaimer in place of this information that reads, "These statements have not been evaluated by the Food and Drug Administration. This product is not intended to diagnose, treat, cure or prevent any disease."

Why are these labels worth discussing? For one, they include information gathered about the treatments during clinical trials.

You can think of them as handy little guides on how your medication affected trial participants, including its uses, interactions, and potential side effects. More importantly, these labels show that publicly available treatments have been evaluated and approved for sale by the FDA. If they haven't, this must be made clear on the label. Also, because an intervention can't be approved by the FDA until it has gone through clinical testing, every single treatment on the market—from medications for chronic illnesses to over-the-counter headache relievers—has been tested on volunteers during clinical trials.

This may not seem like a groundbreaking revelation. But consider the number of FDA-evaluated treatments you use on a regular basis. Each and every one has gone through the entire clinical trials process. Without clinical trials, none of these interventions could have been evaluated for safety or effectiveness. There would be no way of knowing whether these products truly work the way manufacturers claim they do.

If clinical trials ceased to exist, not only would these treatments cease to exist as well, but there would also be the constant risk of snake oil "treatments" making their way back into the market and becoming as common as they once were—a nightmare scenario if there ever was one.

In other words, clinical trials with human participants don't just help us assess the safety and efficacy of new interventions; they are the only way to get new interventions to the public. While alternative testing methods like computer simulation and animal testing are essential to clinical research and trials, they can only do so much to determine how a new treatment or device will work in humans. We must rely on clinical trials—the practical application of clinical research—to help us find new ways to detect, diagnose, and prevent diseases and health conditions.

While the discoveries and advances made through clinical research help benefit the medical community, clinical trials also provide significant benefits to the individuals who volunteer to participate in them. Aside from the satisfaction of knowing that they have aided in the development of potentially life-saving treatments, participants in clinical trials can often expect to receive compensation for their time. Often, they're also receiving the most advanced treatments for their conditions at no cost.

Of course, there is never any guarantee that a standard treatment or a new treatment being tested in a clinical trial will improve a volunteer's condition. But if the new treatment does prove more effective than the standard treatment, participants enrolled in the clinical trial will be the first to benefit.

The bottom line? Clinical trials improve and save lives.

Clinical trials bring new treatments to market

Every doctor wants the same thing: what's best for their patients. But without clinical trials, doctors cannot possibly know what course of treatment is best for each patient. If clinical trials didn't exist, no new drugs, therapies, or medical devices could be developed or brought to market. In this alternate reality, healthcare providers would have no choice but to rely on what's already out there—regardless of whether a better treatment could potentially be developed.

Clinical trials are used to test everything from medications (both over the counter and prescription) and surgical procedures to behavioral therapies and medical devices. Even dietary interventions and educational procedures must be tested before they can be effectively used to improve the daily lives of people around the world. The clinical trial process involves multiple phases, carefully testing every aspect of a drug or device before it's ever allowed in a doctor's office.

The only way that doctors can provide their patients with the most effective treatment options available is to utilize the interventions tested in clinical trials. That's why it's absolutely vital that treatments and products are proven safe and effective before they're made available to patients and healthcare providers. Because we need to be sure that an intervention will work as well as anticipated on humans, we need to actually try them on humans first.

Clinical trials don't just tell us whether a new treatment is more effective than an existing one. They can also determine whether it works better than a placebo or has fewer side effects than the standard treatment option for a given health condition. Clinical trials may even help us discover that a new treatment is safer than existing options, costs less than what's on the market, or is more convenient for patients to use on a regular basis.

One key aspect of clinical trials is that they test newly developed interventions on increasingly large groups of people. If only the first few phases of a trial are successful, for example, this doesn't necessarily mean that the treatment in question will work as intended on a larger population. But if every phase of a trial is successful, then the medication or intervention being tested has a much better chance of acting as intended on the target patient demographic. That's why it's so important that researchers get as many qualified participants as possible for each trial. The more people volunteer for and participate in studies, the more likely researchers are to find meaningful patterns in their data.

For instance, if a new treatment works in 8 out of 10 people (80%), that may sound very promising. However, that sample size (the number of participants being studied) is far too small for researchers to have any confidence about the treatment's effectiveness on a large population. If the treatment works in 800 out of 1,000 people, the success rate remains unchanged, but researchers will have a better idea of how effective the treatment is because these results are more statistically significant. In other words, the chances of 800 people having the same random response to a treatment are much, much lower than the chances of 8 people experiencing the same thing.

Testing for safety and effectiveness

Both doctors and patients want to know with certainty that they are using the most effective treatment for any particular condition. So, if your doctor tells you there are between five and 20 licensed drugs available to treat your condition, how can either of you know which ones are best to try first?

In many cases, patients want to try the drug most likely to effectively treat their condition without causing extreme side effects. While there is no guarantee that a particular treatment will work on any one patient, it makes sense to use the most effective drug with the least potential risks first. After all, the only other option would be trial and error.

Why is trial and error not the best option? Well, a doctor could choose the first drug on the list and write a prescription for it. If it works, that's great. But if it doesn't, the only option is to try the next drug. And if that one fails? Keep moving down the list. Both the doctor and patient would have to work through this process of elimination until chancing upon the medication that works best. This can leave a patient in significant discomfort for a long time, cause unpleasant and potentially dangerous side effects, or allow their condition to progress to a point where more serious intervention is required.

This is exactly what clinical trials were designed to do: eliminate the need for trial-and-error healthcare by systematically testing drugs to determine how well they work in certain patients and situations. Thanks to clinical trials, you and your doctor will know which drugs are most likely to work best as your first course of treatment—and, if that drug doesn't work, which ones are your best alternatives. In other words, clinical trials improve the quality and efficiency of treatment.

Clinical trials also help us determine whether certain drugs work better in particular populations of people. If Drug A works well for men but not for women, for example, a doctor will know to prescribe Drug B for his female patients instead. Or, if Treatment 1 has proven exceptionally effective in Black populations, the doctor might skip Treatment 2 in favor of Treatment 1 for Black patients.

Clinical trials also help medical practitioners weigh the pros and cons of certain treatments. They provide doctors with vital information about the benefits and potential risks or side effects of specific drugs and interventions. As an example, even if a drug is highly effective at treating a particular health condition, severe side effects simply aren't feasible for most patients. A clinical trial may reveal that a novel treatment may lead to unwanted side effects or potential health risks in people taking specific medications, living with certain health conditions, or who are of a certain age.

Ultimately, clinical trials performed under strict supervision are the best way to know if newly developed treatments are safe and effective—especially when administered to specific populations.

Prevention and supportive care

Clinical trials do not always provide cures. Sometimes, they test interventions that prevent health conditions from developing in the first place or help improve overall comfort and quality of life for patients with chronic conditions. In these cases, clinical trials often test more than medications; they may be used to determine the benefits of vaccines, lifestyle changes, educational methods, stress relief techniques, and much more.

These types of clinical trials may, for example, evaluate the efficacy of a newly developed smoking cessation program. Or, they could help determine the measurable effects of mindfulness meditation practices, like yoga, on the physical signs and symptoms of stress.

Preventive trials may also be used to determine health outcomes in people genetically or environmentally predisposed to developing certain health conditions after making lifestyle changes. These trials may, for instance, examine the prevalence of diabetes in a genetically predisposed group of people who eliminate certain foods or start a particular exercise regimen.

Clinical trials help improve the diagnostic process

Clinical trials help doctors and other medical staff more effectively and efficiently diagnose their patients. For one, they allow researchers to identify the characteristic features, signs, and symptoms of health conditions. This lets healthcare providers and diagnosticians know what to look for in their patients when evaluating them for the presence of a health condition, whether based on physical examinations, lab tests, or self-reported symptoms.

The diagnosis of COVID-19 is a fantastic example of this process at work. When the disease was first detected, medical staff instructed patients to look for what they knew to be the characteristic symptoms of the disease: cough and/or fever. However, additional research demonstrated that many COVID-19 patients also lost their senses of taste and smell. Some experienced nausea, stomach cramps, and diarrhea.

In due time, enough clinical trials had been conducted with sufficient numbers of participants that researchers identified six different ways that COVID-19 presents itself. Certain symptoms appeared to present together and were clustered into the following groups:[1]

- "Flu-like" with no fever
- "Flu-like" with fever
- Gastrointestinal
- Severe level 1: fatigue
- Severe level 2: confusion
- Severe level 3: abdominal and respiratory

Identifying these six clusters of symptom presentations allowed doctors to more effectively diagnose COVID-19. It gave them more options when it came to evaluating what a patient might be experiencing based on their symptoms. And as medical professionals successfully identified more cases of COVID-19, they were able to alert infected patients that they should not return to their normal routines because they could potentially infect others with the virus.

This has also opened the door to further research into why people respond to the SARS-CoV-2 virus in different ways, which may eventually provide insights into how we can more effectively treat different individuals with different symptoms.

Most people may not realize that clinical trials actually help many patients receive life-saving diagnoses as a secondary result of the screening process. When an individual is being evaluated as a potential participant in a clinical trial, researchers must determine whether they fit the trial's eligibility criteria. Because each clinical trial has different criteria, candidates may undergo different tests as part of the screening process. The screening process may include health exams, such as blood tests, BMI evaluations, or mammograms. Because of these extensive screenings, many patients discover they have health conditions they were entirely unaware of—conditions that might have gone undiagnosed for years.

At Infinite Clinical Trials, we work with many volunteers who would otherwise be unable to access the extensive testing and health care they receive while participating in a clinical trial. In many cases, these patients are finally able to get the screening and testing they need for free. As a result, they find out for the first time that they have conditions like hepatitis or HIV. While this is never welcome news, it is empowering to play an active role in your healthcare and, after being diagnosed, to have the opportunity to receive the necessary treatment.

One of the most rewarding aspects of running my practice is receiving positive emails from patients thanking us for the opportunity to participate because it may have been years since they've had a full physical. Providing these individuals with the healthcare they need at no cost to them is an invaluable service (and one of the biggest reasons I get up so early to go to work each day).

Clinical trials benefit participants...

Researchers don't design clinical trials with the sole purpose of gathering information. The ultimate purpose of clinical trials is to help the people who participate.

The average doctor may see about 20 patients in a given day if they move quickly and don't get hung up on a complex case. However, hundreds or even thousands of people can participate in a clinical trial. If the treatment being tested is as effective as researchers hope it is, participants stand to gain a lot by receiving the treatment early and at no cost.

Some patients seek out clinical trials because available treatment options haven't worked. They may have seen little to no improvement in their condition, or they may have experienced side effects that rendered their current treatments intolerable. Whatever the case, clinical trials can provide patients with a unique opportunity to explore novel, cutting-edge treatments. They give people suffering from difficult conditions and diseases new hope when all other options have failed.

Even if an experimental treatment isn't as helpful or effective as you would have hoped, you can still take pride in the knowledge that your contributions will advance medical knowledge and ultimately help others. This is why many clinical trials require healthy volunteers (people who do not have the condition being treated but who are willing to contribute to the development of more effective treatments). Researchers use their data as a basis for comparison with volunteers who do have the condition in question.

While these healthy participants may not personally benefit from the intervention being tested, they are helping bring treatments to market for those who truly need them.

...and many more people than just those participating

Clinical trials can also reveal vital information about our relationship to the world around us, such as how a person's environment impacts their health. Past clinical trials have shown that living in underprivileged communities can negatively impact resident medical outcomes. Factors like poverty, poor or unavailable housing, low employment prospects, and racial inequality have all been identified as key factors in determining a person's overall health, as well as their outcomes for certain chronic health conditions.

If people from underprivileged communities never participated in clinical trials, we wouldn't know this. But because they did, medical practitioners, research groups, and even federal and local governments are starting to pay more attention to aiding underprivileged communities. Clinical trials are helping to change policies that have huge influences on public health. Research-based public health initiatives not only ensure that people who need vaccines receive them, but they also equalize access to quality emergency care. Over time, these small changes add up to make a big positive difference.

Furthermore, organizations often allocate research funds based on the results of past clinical trials. When a line of research proves fruitful and produces treatments that are helpful to patients, it proves the validity of the clinical trial model and subsequently encourages more organizations to donate to further research on the topic.

Take cancer, for instance. Clinical trials have proven the usefulness and effectiveness of many cancer-fighting drugs and treatments. However, the success of these trials also shows that more money is needed for further research on different types of cancer and new ways of fighting them. Without additional funding, we will never be able to develop safe, effective strategies for dealing with different types of cancer, and it will take much longer to adopt and distribute effective treatments.

Different groups, different responses to treatment

Within the large groups of people who participate in every clinical trial, there are subgroups. That's why we sometimes find that a new medication works differently in different populations. A treatment may, for instance, be more effective in men than in women, less effective in Black patients than in White ones, or have different effects on patients of different ages.

Because it is so important to test potential treatments and products on all the people they are intended to help, the FDA aims to encourage people of all ages, races, ethnic groups, and genders to participate in clinical trials. Increasing diversity among clinical trial volunteers may demonstrate the effectiveness of a drug across broader populations. It could also help researchers determine the effectiveness of a treatment in very specific populations. Either way, a large and diverse sample size helps us gain knowledge about the different ways that new or existing treatments impact or benefit different types of patients.

As an example, clinical trial researchers have determined that testing new drugs separately in children and adults is critical to developing safer treatments. Children are not just "small adults;" they metabolize compounds differently, and their physiology can vary dramatically depending on their stage of growth. Because their bodies do not always respond to treatments in the same way that adult bodies do, children must undergo separate clinical trials specifically intended for them.

Of course, in most cases, researchers conduct clinical trials on adult participants first. These trials are used to demonstrate the general effectiveness and safety of a treatment, product, or medication. After the safety of the treatment has been confirmed, clinical trials will be conducted on older children, such as teenagers. Finally, if those trials are also successful, researchers will recruit younger children to make sure the treatment is safe for them, too.

Case studies: clinical trials at work

Clinical trials have practical applications across many chronic conditions, acute diseases, and standard medical practices. Here are just two clinical trials that have had real, positive impacts on the lives of many.

Gardasil 9 clinical trial

Human papillomavirus (HPV) is a sexually transmitted viral infection associated with nearly more than 45,000 cancer cases in the United States each year.[2] It is thought to be responsible for more than 90% of all cases of cervical cancer.

Because it is so common, researchers focused on and prioritized the development of a vaccine for HPV. The result was the Gardasil 9 vaccine, which was tested across four clinical trials involving at least 20,500 women between the ages of 16–26. The trials showed that Gardasil 9 completely eliminated cancer caused by certain strains of HPV. It was found to be more than 95% effective in preventing cervical pre-cancers caused by specific strains of HPV in women who had not been previously infected with a targeted HPV type (2vHPV or 4vHPV). Additionally, Gardasil 9 was found to be 96.7% effective in preventing genital pre-cancers in subjects who were not infected at the start of the study and who received all three doses (per the protocol).[3]

Now, the Gardasil 9 vaccine is included in the standard vaccination schedule for all pre-teen children in the United States.

IBCSG-23 for breast cancer

Researchers formed the International Breast Cancer Study Group-23 (IBCSG-23) in order to improve surgical experiences and outcomes for breast cancer patients. Some of the patients in the trial underwent a surgery called axillary dissection, or AD—a procedure in which doctors remove and examine lymph nodes that have been or may be affected by the cancer.

While AD is a procedure with a high success rate, some patients struggle after surgery. Healing can be difficult and painful. Complications may mean postponing further cancer treatments until they are resolved. This can lead to undesirable disease progression and/or chronic pain in affected patients.

In the IBCSG-23 study, some of the patients did not undergo AD. Instead, their doctors treated their cancer without surgical intervention. Researchers watched and tested both groups over time to see if either treatment method had a better outcome.

The results surprised many in the medical community. In certain early-stage breast cancers, AD appeared to cause more harm than good in the study patients. These results led many doctors to stop recommending AD to many breast cancer patients, instead focusing their surgical efforts on those who needed it most.[4]

Denise Flack and Jennifer Waldegrave both participated in this clinical trial. Denise had already watched her mother fight breast cancer and her sister succumb to it. Jennifer was personally battling breast cancer for the second time in her life, and the trial helped her find a successful treatment. Thanks to her participation, her second experience with breast cancer had a much better outcome. Both women agree that the trial saved their lives.

Final thoughts on the importance of clinical trials

In short, clinical trials make people's lives better. They improve health and quality of life by ensuring that safe, effective products are developed to help them feel better, live longer, and even eliminate diseases entirely. Clinical trials are responsible for bringing treatments to market that have improved the lives of millions of people with cancer, heart disease, diabetes, and many other chronic illnesses.

Clinical trials help with everyday conditions, too. Cold medicines, home medical devices (like thermometers), and allergy treatments all undergo extensive testing before your doctor can recommend them or you find them for sale at your local drug store.

Without clinical trials, new medications, products, and treatments would never become available. Even if a few still made it to market, doctors wouldn't have enough information to know how to best use them or for whom they would be most effective. Clinical trials help people live better, work better, and enjoy life more.

PART II

SETTING THE RECORD STRAIGHT

MYTHS AND FACTS ABOUT CLINICAL
TRIALS

THE TRUTH ABOUT CLINICAL TRIALS

Many of us fear the doctor from a young age.

Perhaps it's because of the sterile, uninviting environment. Maybe it's the unfamiliar people poking us here, prodding us there, and asking us highly personal questions. In many cases, it's the uncomfortable procedures we have to sit through (although Mom was right: booster shots really *did* only hurt for a second). Whatever the case, there are many different aspects of medical environments that can make people uneasy.

As we grow older, many of us realize that healthcare providers aren't to be feared, after all. In the vast majority of cases, these people have our health and best interests at heart. After all, many of them have dedicated more than a decade of their lives to learning how to provide medical care—shouldn't they be genuinely invested in helping others?

Still, some of us find that the fears we had as children take on new shapes. They evolve from unease and discomfort to doubt and weariness. They become rooted less in unfamiliarity and uncertainty and more so in disappointment and dissatisfaction.

As women, many of us have seen healthcare providers undervalue or dismiss our pain.[1] And as African Americans, many of us have received a lesser quality of care than our peers.[2] No matter who you are, it's the regrettable reality that healthcare is not always as fair as it should be. Doctors are people; people are flawed. And no matter how kind or well-meaning, anyone can be influenced by unconscious bias.

It's understandable, then, that some people are uncomfortable with the idea of participating in clinical trials. Their residual fears of the doctor (*clinical, sterile, unfamiliar, painful*) and newer fears of dismissal or inadequate treatment carry over. These fears inform their perceptions of clinical trials—another arm of what they understand to be an unpleasant (if not outright unjust) healthcare system. Volunteering for a trial, then, would be nothing more than an unnecessary burden. After all, if we wouldn't willingly visit the doctor without needing to, why would we subject ourselves to something seen as similarly unpleasant when we have every right not to?

Well, first of all, that's the great thing: you have every right to choose not to participate in clinical trials. It's entirely up to you. At the core of clinical trials is the principle of consent—the notion that study participants are willing volunteers who have donated their time of their own accord, only after being informed of everything a clinical trial entails.

I stand firmly by the fact that no one has to participate in a clinical trial if they aren't interested in (or comfortable with) doing so. But I'm equally partial to the idea that no one should rule out volunteering until they understand clinical trials as best they can. That doesn't mean devoting years of your life to learning the ins and outs of healthcare legislation, regulatory practices, and scientific methods. After all, it would be unrealistic (and unfair) to expect every participant in a clinical trial to do so. It does, however, mean taking the time to understand what clinical trials are—and what they are not. As in all areas of life, gathering all the evidence and information you need to understand clinical trials is the best thing you can do before making a decision on them—one way or the other.

In the context of this book, the educational process starts with dissecting and reframing the misunderstandings surrounding clinical trials. While I sometimes refer to these misunderstandings as "myths," I can't simply discount all of them as blatant lies that have been pulled from thin air. As with any misunderstandings, they arose from somewhere real—be it fear, falsehoods, a lack of information, or historical injustices.

Yes—there are many origins of the myths surrounding clinical trials. Some have come from genuine misunderstanding or lack of information about clinical trials and the processes surrounding them. Others have developed in response to insidious experiments that have been conducted posing as "clinical trials." (As we've discussed, the history of human medical trials has not always been an ethical one. While clinical trials themselves are transparent, regulated, and always put human safety at the forefront, some researchers have not adhered to these tenets, targeting people of color, in particular, as subjects of these deplorable experiments). And some misunderstandings come from somewhere in the middle.

It's particularly important to note that clinical trials don't always receive positive press. The resulting medical breakthroughs themselves frequently make the news. This was especially true, as we saw, when the race to develop COVID-19 vaccines was in full swing. This process was chronicled in nearly real time—it seemed like every day, different front-page headlines detailed recent developments and the newest, most promising options. But the unfortunate fact is that, in the average year, one doesn't typically hear about the clinical trials responsible for the front-page medical breakthroughs. If you do hear about clinical trials in the media, it is often only when something has gone wrong.

While my wish is that clinical trials start to receive the full credit (or, at least, positive recognition) they deserve, this will not happen overnight. This is, in part, why I am writing this book. My goal isn't only to equip you with knowledge about clinical trials, but also to explain the importance of clinical trials in advancing medical knowledge and human health.

Perhaps most importantly, it's crucial to understand that in virtually all cases, these myths come from people who have never participated in clinical trials. They haven't come from people who have had bad experiences with studies, but from those who have not volunteered because of any of the above reasons.

In fact, many of the people who have participated in clinical trials choose not to share this fact for fear that they will be ostracized by those who incorrectly assume such myths to be true. This is particularly true of Black Americans, as ethicality and fair treatment, particularly in medicine, have always been of concern to us. To trust the healthcare industry (and, by extension, the government) is seen as the ultimate act of relinquishing our bodies to the institutions that have repeatedly betrayed us. Clearly, this is a complex issue. It will be no simple feat to sway those who have already made up their minds about the motivations of scientists, pharmaceutical companies, and even others like myself in the clinical trials industry. But no matter how difficult, these misunderstandings need to be addressed.

In the following chapters, I hope to help shed some light on the most common "myths" about clinical research (and clinical trials, in particular). If I help at least one reader understand clinical trials better, I'll have met the goal I set out to achieve in writing this book.

And even if you are already interested in participating in clinical trials, chances are, you still have some questions. I hope I'll be able to help you, as well. You may even realize you've believed some of these myths to be true.

"CLINICAL TRIAL VOLUNTEERS ARE MISTREATED."

The myth that clinical trial volunteers are not just treated unfairly but actually mistreated or misled is a common one. The reality is that this couldn't be further from the truth.

It's not just anecdotal experience that has shown me that clinical trial participants are treated with responsibility and compassion—it's also the fact that years' worth of work and legislation have been dedicated to protecting their rights, privacy, and, above all, safety.

Without engaged, consenting participants, clinical trials would cease to exist. If clinical trials today were to routinely exploit or take advantage of participants in any way, people would simply stop volunteering. It's the job of clinical researchers and trial coordinators to ensure that volunteers and potential participants feel as comfortable, confident, and well-informed as possible throughout the entire process of participating in a trial.

Everyone involved in clinical trials, from sponsors and researchers to clinical trial practices and participants, shares the same common goal: to further medical knowledge in order to make people's lives better. And it is the participants in clinical trials that are to thank for volunteering their time and efforts.

For this alone, they have earned clinical researchers' and trial coordinators' full respect and transparency.

Myth: "Clinical trial volunteers are treated like 'human guinea pigs' or 'lab rats.'"

Most of us are familiar with the term "human guinea pig." It evokes dreadful images: fearful, unwilling test subjects forced into hellish experiments led by mad scientists. Or, perhaps, it conjures a picture of something a little less animated: a secretive government being paid off by greedy pharmaceutical companies to allow the testing of potentially unsafe drugs on humans.

Whatever the case, the term "human guinea pig" denotes a few core ideas: unwillingness (on the part of the participants), dishonesty (from those running the experiment), and danger (unsafe or questionable medications or treatments). Above all, it implies a lack of physical autonomy—that by deciding to participate in a clinical trial, you are relinquishing your right to say what is done to your body. This is, perhaps, the most frightening prospect of all.

Fact: Strict guidelines are put in place to ensure that you and all other volunteers are treated safely, fairly, and ethically.

The image of a lab rat being strapped to a table and poked, prodded, or otherwise experimented upon against its will could not be further from the experiences people have during clinical trials. Participants in clinical trials are human subjects. As such, they are treated like just that: humans.

Clinical researchers and coordinators work hard to protect and respect participants' rights. They treat volunteers with all the dignity and integrity that should be expected of any type of medical professional. And, above all, they understand that your body is yours: only you can have the final say in what is done to you.

As such, researchers, clinicians, and coordinators ask for your permission before each blood draw, lab test, X-ray, or any other type of procedure performed during a trial. While you will be made aware of each of these procedures before the trial even begins, those performing them will take care to ensure that you understand what is happening—and, more importantly, why it is being done—every step of the way. This is, as we will soon explore in more detail, all part of maintaining what's known as *informed consent* throughout the entirety of the clinical trial.

Unlike guinea pigs, lab rats, or other images of involuntary medical experimentation, individuals who volunteer to participate in clinical trials do so on a completely consensual basis. No one will ever force you to participate in a clinical trial, no matter how important or beneficial the intervention being studied is anticipated to be. What's more, no one will ever force you to stay in a trial if you are no longer comfortable with it—even if you have signed a consent form and the trial has already begun. You are free to leave at any time because you are volunteering to participate—not surrendering your rights and autonomy (the ability to make personal decisions for yourself) in the name of science.

If you are unsure whether individual researchers, clinicians, or coordinators can be trusted to uphold the highest standards when it comes to your rights and autonomy, understand that such concerns are, to put it lightly, a big deal when it comes to human trials. Dedicated governmental and international agencies, commissions, and oversight boards exist with the sole purpose of ensuring that clinical studies are performed according to strict moral and ethical parameters. Researchers are subject to such regulations from the moment they begin recruiting participants to the end of a study (and, in many cases, long after it's completed).

Additionally, clinical trials' protocols (the documents outlining each and every one of the procedures involved) are reviewed by panels called research ethics boards (REBs) or institutional review boards (IRBs). These panels, which consist of researchers, doctors, and laymen (members of the general public), conduct oversight and review to ensure that every study is properly designed, legally compliant, and ethically sound and does not subject participants to unnecessary or overly severe risks. It can, at times, be a long process for a trial to obtain approval from the several different committees responsible for doing so. It's not at all uncommon for it to take years for a clinical trial to go from conception to the first steps of patient recruitment. But we would much rather take the time to ensure that a trial is sound than run the risk of sacrificing participants' safety and rights—even if it meant speeding up the approval process.

The same level of oversight and responsibility is maintained throughout a trial once it has begun. If a patient is to undergo any sort of test or procedure during a study (including one considered as routine and benign as an imaging test, like a CT scan), it must first be approved by a committee. The same is true even if the exam is part of your routine care. Though they may, at times, seem redundant or overly cautious, these regulations, panels, and oversight measures all exist to protect the rights and inherent autonomy of clinical trial participants. The practices used to maintain respect and transparency between clinical researchers and participants are constantly evolving to uphold and improve the ethical integrity we've spent years establishing in this industry.

Myth: "By participating in a clinical trial, I'll have to give up some (or all) of my privacy."

As we progress further into the digital age, many of us are becoming more concerned about our privacy. Credit card numbers, bank account passwords, and personally identifying information—all of it is up for grabs if we're not careful enough.

Given the prevalence of these concerns, it's not surprising

that many people participating in clinical trials question how their medical histories will be handled. Many people wonder, "If the information gathered from a study is surveyed by multiple agencies and teams and used to bring new treatments to market, couldn't my information be made public, or at least used in ways I'm not comfortable with?"

That's a valid question. It's a good sign that so many people take their health history and privacy so seriously. One of the best things you can do when considering whether to participate in a clinical trial is to ask questions and gather as much knowledge as you need to feel one hundred percent sure of your decision. But before delving into the details of how clinical trials are set up to protect patient privacy, I think it's worth exploring the concept of privacy in relation to medical research (and the healthcare industry as a whole).

To do so, we will look to an invaluable book: *Beyond the HIPAA Privacy Rule: Enhancing Privacy, Improving Health Through Research.*[1] In the second chapter, "The Value and Importance of Health Information Privacy," it is explained that concepts of privacy, in the context of personal information, are closely intertwined with those of confidentiality and security. These three concepts, however, are distinctly different from each other.

Privacy, it explains, addresses the question of who has access to personal information and under what conditions. It is concerned with the collection, storage, and use of this information, as well as how data collected for one purpose can be used for another (if it can be used for another purpose at all). One of the largest concerns surrounding the concept of privacy is whether an individual has given others the authority to use his or her personal information in certain ways.

Confidentiality, on the other hand, refers to the safeguarding of information gathered in the context of an intimate relationship (just like that between a researcher and patient, as this relationship is formed on mutual trust and transparency). It deals with how the information exchanged in such a relationship (patient information) is protected. In the context of healthcare, confidentiality is the principle that prevents medical professionals from disclosing any information shared with them in patient-physician relationships to others (as this would constitute a breach of confidentiality).

Security is described, in part, as the measures necessary for preventing unauthorized access, modification, use, and sharing of personal information. These measures help protect personal information from unauthorized use or distribution.

The chapter goes on to explore the many reasons why the medical community places such value on the privacy, confidentiality, and security of patients' health information. In a more philosophical sense, some individuals have considered privacy to be an essential part of our well-being. More practically speaking, privacy's importance arises from its promotion of other fundamental human values, including personal autonomy, individuality, respect, and dignity and worth as human beings. These values are fundamental to ethical clinical trials, but what would happen if these concepts weren't respected or safeguarded?

The disclosure of personally identifiable health information can have a variety of negative consequences, ranging from embarrassment (at best) to discrimination (at worst). Say, for example, that you have a congenital (from birth) heart defect and work in a physically demanding industry, such as construction or moving. Were your employer to see your personal health information (and, as a result, learn about your heart defect), they may question whether you could continue to perform your job —regardless of whether or not your condition impacts your overall health or your ability to work.

Conversely, maintaining privacy when it comes to personal health can have huge positive impacts—namely, it can vastly improve patient-provider relationships. Knowing that your healthcare provider (or, in this case, your clinical trial team) is taking all necessary precautions to safeguard your privacy affords you the confidence that the information you share with them will remain secure. This can help promote more open, effective communication between patients and doctors—a practice that's essential to providing high-quality care and ensuring patients' autonomy. In other words, when you are confident that the concerns you share with your healthcare team will remain private, you can give them all the information they need to provide you with the best possible care.

It's important to understand that, at the end of the day, "privacy" means different things to different people. While one person may expect their health information to be kept private at all costs, another person may be comfortable with non-identifying information being used to further medical knowledge.

For example, a review of 43 national surveys on healthy privacy conducted from 1993 to 2007 revealed just how disparate patients' concerns about their health information could be. In some of the surveys, the majority of respondents said they were not comfortable with their health information being provided for the purpose of health research, except with notice and express consent. In other surveys, however, a majority responded that they would be willing to forgo such notice and consent, provided that certain safeguards would be in place and their information would be used for specific types of research. A more recent poll, for instance, found that 63% of respondents would provide general consent for the use of their medical records for the purpose of research if they were guaranteed that no personally identifiable health information would be released.[2] Interestingly enough, this is similar to the percentage of people who reported being willing to participate in a "clinical research study."[3]

The fact is, however, that no matter how concerned you are with the privacy, confidentiality, and security of your personal information, healthcare providers—and, of course, clinical trial teams—take these concepts extremely seriously and utilize every measure needed to uphold them.

. . .

Fact: Researchers must keep any identifying information about you private. Patient confidentiality is key to conducting high-quality, ethically run clinical trials.

One important (but less well-known) benefit of clinical trials is that they provide researchers with a wealth of valuable information about human health. This information isn't simply discarded after a trial has finished. Instead, the information gathered from clinical trials is often used to carry out secondary research—a research method that involves using already existing data to inform new investigations.

When a scientist draws on past knowledge to contextualize or support their findings, they are using secondary research to supplement their own. If, for instance, a researcher wanted to investigate the features of a musculoskeletal disorder with the aim of developing a new, more effective treatment than those already on the market, they would start by gathering existing materials with information on the disorder and its current standard treatments. This would provide them with the background information needed to guide their research and direct them toward finding new solutions. Such secondary research can provide scientists with insights into previous researchers' methods and approaches for treating the disorder. It also allows them to identify gaps in science's current understanding of the disorder or its treatments and hopefully fill them with their findings.

But the information the researcher takes from these studies is based on data obtained from real people. It isn't just numbers or arbitrarily created facts and figures—in this case, it represents facts about real individuals with a certain disorder. So, how can it be that researchers are allowed to divulge personal health information on such public platforms for all to access? Wouldn't this be a breach of privacy, confidentiality, and security?

You may recall my mention in Chapter 2 of the "Common

Rule"—a set of ethical requirements put in place to protect participants in biomedical and behavioral research. Within this policy are guidelines governing exactly how to handle health information obtained from human subjects to be used in secondary research. Thanks to the Common Rule, researchers take particular precautions to protect the identities of the individuals that have provided them with health information and data. This is done through a process called "de-identification." This process involves removing all patient information associated with a person's health data, from their date of birth and laboratory test results to their gender and race.[4]

While there are a few different approaches to de-identification, the process generally involves presenting data so as to render it virtually or entirely not individually identifiable. In other words, this process prevents anyone who is accessing information through secondary research from tracing any one piece of data back to an individual participant (or from identifying an individual based on their data in combination with others').

While processes like these afford patients privacy and confidentiality, there are still some complexities regarding the use of health data collected through clinical trials. While it's one of the primary goals of researchers and clinical trial teams to protect patients' personal privacy, the health information gathered during clinical studies can provide valuable insights and immense benefits to society as a whole. It can be used to inform and facilitate the development of groundbreaking new therapies, diagnostic techniques, and more.

Clearly, a delicate balance must be struck between security and potential medical advancement. While keeping patients' personal health information secure is of the utmost importance, researchers must also be allowed to use the information they have collected to improve medical knowledge and health outcomes. Although it's not specific to clinical trials, there is a policy that strikes just that balance: the HIPAA Standards for

Privacy of Individually Identifiable Health Information (referred to as the "Privacy Rule").

As stated by the U.S. Department of Health and Human Services, a major goal of the Privacy Rule is to "assure that individuals' health information is properly protected while allowing the flow of health information needed to provide and promote high quality health care and to protect the public's health and well being."[5] It aims to permit the use of important health information in a way that best protects the rights and privacy of "people who seek care and healing."

This rule established, for the first time, a set of national standards for the protection of private medical information (called "protected health information"). It outlines the ways in which certain organizations can use and disclose this information and establishes standards regarding individuals' privacy and rights—in particular, their rights to understand and control how their health information is used.

As for clinical trials, in particular, the informed consent document and process are key to outlining all precautions and considerations taken into account regarding patient data during a clinical trial. Before enrolling in a trial, the FDA requires that a potential participant receive a statement (usually found in the informed consent document) describing the confidentiality of the information to be collected during the trial, how identifying records will be kept, and the possibility that the FDA may inspect these records. This portion of an informed consent document may also include a statement giving you the option to authorize the release of any significant findings about your health (or the fact that you are participating in the study) to your family doctor or primary healthcare provider.

Ultimately, upholding privacy, confidentiality, and security when it comes to patient information gathered in clinical trials is both legally required and ethically necessary. In some cases, special consideration is even taken for patient confidentiality (when, for instance, dealing with individuals who may be considered "vulnerable subjects," including children and those who are critically or terminally ill). All of this serves the purpose of protecting patients' rights, affording them the respect and understanding they deserve, and preserving their inherent right to autonomy.

Final thoughts on the rights of clinical trial volunteers

Modern clinical trials are forged in consent and ethicality, not deception and exploitation. They are designed to protect your rights as an individual and ensure that you understand what is happening and what you are being asked to do every step of the way. While images of the lab rat or guinea pig are commonly misunderstood as representative of patients' experiences in human studies, they are fortunately not representative of the reality of modern clinical trials.

It is not just our legal obligation to follow certain protocols, adhere to certain rules and regulations, and take certain measures to protect patients' rights. It is, over all else, our moral and ethical responsibility to do so. These are not arbitrary requirements or overly strict mandates, and I do not see them as burdensome. Instead, I view them as the reflection of countless people's tireless efforts to put into law what we want for all our patients: transparency, fairness, and respect.

"PARTICIPATING IN CLINICAL TRIALS IS EXPENSIVE."

Another one of the most common concerns I hear from people interested in participating in clinical trials is that they won't be able to afford to do so. Many people believe that the costs associated with clinical trials are high—particularly those associated with medical testing, transportation, and the treatment itself. Aside from these concerns, patients (especially those of low income or with little job security) often fear that clinical trials will require them to miss so much work that their income will be disrupted, or they will have to find long-term childcare. Add in the fact that many people turn to clinical trials to access treatments they couldn't otherwise afford, and cost is a natural concern. These worries are normal. In fact, very few people have no questions about costs before beginning clinical trials.

The truth is, clinical trials are expensive—but not for the patients participating in them. According to a study on clinical trials from 2016, the average cost of a phase 1 clinical study ranged from $1.4 to $6.6 million, while phase 3 studies cost anywhere from $11.5 to $52.9 million.[1] There are many factors that go into these high price tags. Patient recruitment, clinical supplies and equipment, and monitoring participants for safety are just some of the expenses that must be accounted for while conducting a clinical trial. And while efforts are being made to bring the costs of clinical trials down, bearing the burden of these expenses ultimately lies on trial sponsors and research teams—not participants.

At my practice (and at many others), patients pay nothing out of pocket to participate in clinical trials. In fact, they're often compensated for their time and reimbursed for expenses like the cost of transportation. After all, these volunteers are helping to shape the future of healthcare. They deserve to receive proper thanks for the time and effort they've dedicated.

Here, we'll take a look at some of the prevailing myths about the costs associated with clinical trials. While you should always check in with a clinical trials coordinator about the particulars of a trial, these are true for my practice, Infinite Clinical Trials, and for the majority of practices across the United States.

Myth: "The out-of-pocket costs associated with clinical trials are extremely high."

If you've been diagnosed with a chronic or serious medical condition or illness, you understand just how stressful it can be. Perhaps the standard treatments your doctor has provided haven't worked, or they've caused so many side effects that they aren't feasible for you. Or, perhaps, you've been struggling to pay the costs associated with your care and feel like you've simply run out of options. So, after considering the possibility of volunteering for a clinical trial, you decide to investigate a particular study near you.

As it turns out, you qualify for the trial and pass its screening process (more on that later). But maybe you have a health insurance plan with a high deductible or significant copays that you have to cover each time you see a medical provider. Given the expenses already associated with your health condition, the thought of adding more costs to your baseline care might make participating in a clinical trial seem impossible.

What's more, you've heard that clinical trials often involve additional testing, medication, or monitoring on top of what you're already receiving. Wouldn't that just be an additional financial burden?

Fact: Most trial costs are covered by the trial itself.

Put simply, there are no out-of-pocket costs associated with participating in clinical trials.

All costs associated with clinical trials conducted in the United States are funded in one of two ways: by private businesses (such as pharmaceutical companies or medical research foundations) or, in some cases, by the federal government (through institutions such as the National Institutes of Health or the National Cancer Institute).

As we already know, if a pharmaceutical company produces a new drug, devises a new treatment method, or designs a new medical device, they must first have it approved for consumer sale and distribution. While the government and multiple advisory boards approve and oversee such trials, the money used to fund the trials comes from the drug company itself.

In other cases, researchers are looking to test new treatments or interventions. They receive funding for their trials in the form of grants. These grants, which may come from government institutions or private sponsors (including pharmaceutical companies), are used to cover all costs associated with these trials. Organizations dedicated to eradicating certain types of cancer, for instance, often raise money for research and testing of new treatments and modes of prevention.

But the bottom line is that no matter where its funding comes from, the medical costs directly associated with a clinical trial are paid for with these resources—not by volunteers. If you are taking part in a trial to test a newly developed drug, for instance, external resources will be used to cover the cost of the drug, as well as any expenses associated with the facility where you receive the drug, the personnel who administer the drug and monitor your health, and any testing whose sole purpose is to collect data about the drug.

But what about any routine care for your condition that you receive during a trial? What if, for instance, you must receive a monthly blood test to check your liver function while taking a particular medication?

In many cases, these will be covered by your health insurance.[2] In fact, federal law requires that most insurance providers cover the costs of routine healthcare visits and procedures that take place during an approved clinical trial. This may include anything from routine blood work and scans to radiology tests— even if it's part of your normal care. As long as a procedure or test is being performed to check on your general health during a trial, your insurance must cover it. (Conversely, if a clinical trial requires additional blood work or lab testing to check on the potential side effects of a treatment, the drug company or trial sponsor will cover the costs, rather than your insurance provider.)

It's true that a few requirements must be met in order for your insurance company to cover a test or procedure. At a private clinical trials practice such as mine, however, these requirements—including the requirements that a clinical trial receives approval from an institutional review board (IRB) and that the participant qualifies for the trial—are met from the start. As a result, in most cases, your insurance will cover procedures or testing incidental to the trial you're participating in. But one of the best parts about participating in a clinical trial is the fact that insurance is not required to participate. Regardless of coverage status, clinical trials allow individuals to receive top-of-the-line treatments and expert medical care at no cost.

. . .

Myth: Travel expenses, childcare, and other associated costs of participation are the patient's sole responsibility.

Even after your concerns about the costs of medical care are addressed, you may worry about the other expenses associated with participating in a clinical trial, such as those involved in getting you to and from the trial facilities.

Many trials require you to visit certain facilities in order to receive the experimental treatment and be carefully monitored for its effects on you and your health. In some cases, this facility may be relatively close to you, such as a local hospital or lab. At other times, you may be required to travel to the researcher's location. Some clinical trials, for instance, take place at large research facilities like Johns Hopkins in Maryland, the Mayo Clinic in Minnesota, or the Cleveland Clinic in Ohio.

No matter how long a clinical trial lasts, the frequency of these in-person visits can vary. They may only occur once or twice over the course of the trial, or they may be required at regular intervals, such as once or more per week. Additionally, the length of time you spend at each facility can fluctuate, with some visits taking a couple of hours and others requiring inpatient stays of several days at a time.

As you'd expect, attending every visit will require certain expenses, whether you are driving, taking a bus across town, or purchasing plane tickets to travel across the country. Especially in the case of overnight stays, you'll also need to consider the costs of meals, hotel stays (for yourself and for anyone accompanying you), childcare and/or pet care costs, and more. And if a trial requires you to take regular trips at different times of the year, you may not feel confident in your ability to accurately predict how much each trip will cost.

With all these costs considered, participating in a clinical trial may seem too expensive—even if you know that all of the medical costs themselves will be covered. Luckily, these additional expenses are accounted for by clinical trial teams.

· · ·

Fact: Many clinical trials offer reimbursement programs that cover most (or all) associated costs.

As explained above, clinical trials are funded in one of two ways: by private companies or by third-party sponsors. In order to incentivize participation, many of these sponsors set aside a portion of the funds allocated toward a clinical trial to help volunteers cover the extra costs associated with participating.

These programs are usually set up on a reimbursement basis. This means that you will pay for things like travel and childcare upfront, then submit your receipts (often using a particular form) to request reimbursement after the fact. The time it takes to receive your reimbursement can vary, depending on the trial you're participating in and its unique policies and procedures. Ultimately, however, if your trial has a reimbursement program, you will be compensated for much of your travel and other associated costs.

It's important to be aware of the fact that some clinical trials don't advertise their reimbursement programs. You can (and should) always ask whether a particular trial reimburses participants for associated costs—and if they do, which particular costs are eligible for reimbursement. If trials have limited funding, they may set a cap on how much reimbursement participants can receive, or they may reimburse some expenses (like the cost of plane tickets) but not others (like the costs associated with childcare or pet care while you are out of town).

Make sure you take full advantage of any reimbursement programs that clinical trials offer. Utilizing these programs does much, much more than help you cover the costs of participating in a trial. It also demonstrates to researchers and sponsors that reimbursement programs help motivate people to participate in clinical trials and that these programs are an important part of making trial participation more accessible.

As an additional incentive, some clinical trials offer stipends in place of (or in addition to) reimbursement programs. These stipends can take multiple forms: you may receive a certain amount of money for each month of your participation in a trial or every time you receive a treatment or complete a medical test. Other trials may simply pay a stipend to participants upon the completion of the trial. If you participate in a clinical trial that offers these types of incentives, you will receive the stipend regardless of your travel expenses and other associated costs. While you can spend your stipend money on anything that you wish, many volunteers use it to partially or totally offset things like travel or childcare costs. This is just another way that clinical research teams help reduce any potential stresses that may arise while participating in a clinical trial.

Myth: Participating in a clinical trial will require me to miss too much time at work.

Now, you understand how the medical costs associated with a clinical trial are covered. You also know that you won't have to pay out of pocket for travel and other trial-related costs. For many people, however, an additional concern remains: they simply cannot afford to miss work in order to participate in a clinical trial, no matter how much compensation they receive or how promising the experimental treatment is.

If you are working while dealing with a chronic or serious medical condition, it can be challenging enough to complete your job's responsibilities even without participating in a clinical trial. You may be so tired from making appointments and undergoing regular testing that it becomes difficult to complete job-related tasks, or you may be experiencing treatment-related side effects that make everyday responsibilities more challenging than they were before. You might even feel that you are already out of the office quite a bit as a result of navigating your health condition.

Given the time it can take to receive trial-related tests and treatments (and the ways these may affect you), you might be questioning whether you'd be able to keep up with your job and participate in a trial at the same time.

Even if your employer is generous and supportive of you as you find effective treatments, they can only give you so much paid leave over the course of any given year. If a particular clinical trial requires a great deal of travel, you may be concerned about maxing out your paid time off and having to take unpaid days in order to complete the trial. And if you have medical insurance through your job, you may face the added anxiety of losing it (and all of the medical coverage associated with it) if you were forced to cut your hours or quit your job entirely.

So, how do clinical trials account for those with responsibilities to their jobs?

Fact: Most clinical trials will work with you so you can stay employed.

Most clinical researchers and coordinators are realists. They understand that you need to keep your job in order to cover the costs of living and your standard healthcare. They also know that you are most likely not willing to risk your income, financial well-being, and insurance coverage just to be part of a clinical trial, no matter how promising it may be.

Because of this, many clinical trials teams do their best to accommodate participants' work schedules. Some will work with you to locate trial sites whose schedules are compatible with yours or even limit extended trial-related trips when you are running out of vacation days and/or sick leave. Others will go as far as to offer treatment times outside of normal business hours —even potentially working weekends—so that you can fully participate while remaining employed.

The best thing you can do is what I always aim to facilitate at my practice: talk to clinical trial coordinators about how you can make a trial work with your schedule. You'd be surprised at how accommodating many of them are. After all, because so many clinical trials need more eligible participants, study coordinators will often do everything they can to accommodate your needs and your schedule.

The bottom line is this: you should never have to risk losing your job, income, or insurance coverage in order to participate in a clinical trial. If these are concerns of yours, bring them up with those running the clinical trial, and be sure to get all your questions answered before you agree to participate.

Final thoughts on the costs of clinical trials

Clinical trials are expensive to conduct, but participants should not have to foot the bill.

More and more clinical trials teams and sponsors are making every effort to keep research-associated costs out of participants' pockets. When it comes to medical expenses, they do this by providing medication and trial-associated testing free of cost and by working with your insurance company to make sure you are covered for all testing and procedures you receive while enrolled in a trial.

Clinical trial coordinators are also working hard to prevent other trial-related costs, such as travel, accommodations, and childcare, from burdening participants. Reimbursement programs often allow participants to recoup what they've spent to participate in a clinical trial, while stipends afford participants the opportunity to offset trial costs and receive compensation for their time.

Research teams also make every effort to allow participants to continue working their jobs as usual while participating in clinical trials. They may offer treatments and tests outside of regular business hours or allow you to receive treatment and testing at a location that is easier for you to access from work.

While it may seem too good to be true that groundbreaking

medical interventions could be available to patients at no cost (or even to your financial betterment), the exciting reality is that it's not. Researchers and coordinators understand that committing your time and efforts to participate in a clinical trial is invaluable. Worrying about the costs of receiving medical care should be the least of your concerns.

MYTHS ABOUT INFORMED CONSENT

There's a reason that this chapter isn't titled like the rest: there is no one prevailing myth about informed consent. While the most common misconception is the first one addressed in this chapter ("Informed consent is just a piece of paper I have to read and sign"), there are so many different aspects to informed consent that no single myth sufficiently addresses them.

If you're thinking of participating in a clinical trial, it's vital that you understand what informed consent is, how it works, and what role you will play in the process. It's my opinion (and the opinion of many other professionals in my field) that informed consent is one of the most important components of a clinical trial. In many ways, it exists at the heart of the clinical trials process—it helps ensure clear communication and patient understanding from start to finish.

Informed consent can be thought of as the culmination of years' worth of considerations about ethicality, good clinical practice, patient involvement and understanding, and, of course, patient consent. Its purpose is much, much greater than just to confirm that a participant has been informed of the risks involved with participating in a clinical trial. Rather, informed consent is a process. It's the means by which participants are made to understand all aspects of a clinical trial to the fullest extent possible.

Myth: "Informed consent is just a piece of paper I have to read and sign."

It's true that informed consent is, in part, a document. The purpose of an informed consent document is to provide patients with all the information they need in order to make a confident, well-informed decision on whether or not to participate in a particular clinical trial.

People unfamiliar with clinical trials (and informed consent, in particular) often believe that patient education begins and ends with such a document. But an informed consent document alone cannot guarantee a patient's full understanding of a clinical trial—it's just one aspect of a larger educational process.

Fact: The informed consent document is just one part of the ongoing educational process that makes up informed consent.

Informed consent involves two essential pieces: the document itself and the process of informed consent. Clinical trial researchers and coordinators know that a physical document alone likely won't be enough for you to understand the entire scope of what participating in a particular clinical trial means. Because of this, informed consent is not a one-time informational session that ends in you signing on the dotted line. In actuality, it's an ongoing, interactive discussion.

This discussion, which comprises the bulk of the informed consent process, provides you with continuous explanations of all aspects of the clinical trial. This is done with the purpose of helping you make an educated decision about whether to begin participating (or continue to participate) in a clinical trial.

But providing information to patients isn't the only important part of this process. Informed consent also requires clinical trial researchers and coordinators to facilitate potential participants' understanding of all the information that's been presented to them. In other words, it's not enough for them to simply give the information to potential volunteers—they must also take the time to make sure that this information is fully understood. This involves allowing individuals to ask questions about anything they don't understand. In fact, potential participants and enrolled volunteers alike must be given sufficient opportunities to learn about a trial and read the consent document thoroughly enough that they understand it entirely, as well as ask questions about anything they're unsure about.

While the informed consent document serves the purpose of obtaining "initial consent," the overarching goal of the informed consent process is to obtain what's known as "continued consent." Continued consent refers to the responsibility of clinical trial researchers and coordinators to obtain ongoing, repeated consent from trial participants. In other words, they must make sure that patients still understand and consent to all aspects of a trial—even after it has begun, and regardless of whether a patient gave consent upon enrolling. This "re-consent" is obtained at various intervals throughout a clinical trial as legally required and as ethically necessary.

Myth: "Informed consent only tells me about the risks or dangers of participating in a trial."

Even if you understand all the potential risks involved in a clinical trial, that by no means tells you everything you need to know about it. While this is an important part of making a well-informed decision about whether to participate, it's certainly not the only one.

Informed consent doesn't just provide the worst-case scenario. It also explains all other aspects of a study, helping you make a decision about whether it's worth participating in and understand what to expect when enrolling.

Fact: Informed consent—both the document and the process —covers all aspects of a clinical trial.

Informed consent addresses a broad scope of information about a clinical trial—much more than just its potential risks. It details all the information you'll need to make a decision about whether to participate. So, what information does it cover, exactly?

The informed consent document itself outlines the potential risks involved in a trial. To this end, it presents all known information about the safety, applications, and potential effectiveness of the intervention being tested. While the goal of clinical trials is to benefit patients by getting promising new treatments approved for market, the FDA requires that an informed consent document inform participants of a number of facts: that they may not benefit from the clinical trial, that they may be exposed to unknown risks, and that they are entering into a study that may be very different from the standard medical practices that they currently know. In addition to presenting the informed consent document, clinical trial researchers and coordinators will make sure that patients understand exactly what these risks are, whether they might impact certain individuals differently from others, and how the potential risks of a particular trial stack up against its potential benefits.

But informed consent provides so much more information than this. In short, it must advise potential and enrolled participants of the purpose and details of a clinical trial. This includes general information, such as a statement explaining that the study involves research, an explanation of the purposes of this research, and any potential benefits that may be expected to result from it. It also includes more specific information that you'll need while planning ahead for a trial, such as the exact number of visits you'll need to make time for, the types and durations of each procedure that will be performed (and any potential discomforts associated with them), and for how long the clinical trial is expected to last.

It's important to understand that informed consent documents are written so that the average person can understand them. It's not the goal of clinical researchers or trial coordinators to trick you into signing something you don't fully comprehend. For this reason, researchers don't just have to obtain consent—they have to do so in ways that are meaningful to the people giving it. In fact, researchers have even tested different consent forms to determine which are the most comprehensive and easiest to understand for potential research subjects.[1] If you don't understand a consent document, someone must explain it to you so that you feel confident in what you are agreeing to. And if you would like to take the time to review it on your own, you can ask for a copy of a trial's consent document at any time.

Clinical trials are not scary or malevolent. There is so much more to them than just their potential risks. That's exactly why the informed consent process and document provide potential participants with a breadth of information—they need to know all the particulars of a trial, not just any possible risks, before deciding whether to enroll.

Myth: "Once I enroll, I won't be able to change my mind and leave a clinical trial."

So, you've decided to enroll in a clinical trial. You've discussed the details of the study with coordinators and ensured that you could commit the time to make each visit. You're excited about the potential benefits of the treatment being tested.

The trial begins, and within a few weeks, you start to feel dizzy and lightheaded—potential side effects that you learned about before signing your informed consent document. While mild and not unusual, you decided before enrolling that you'd stop participating in the trial if you experienced any noticeable side effects. But there's a problem: you've already signed the informed consent document.

You may be thinking: "Doesn't that mean I'm obligated to continue participating in the trial? After all, I was made aware of these potential side effects and had every opportunity to consider the potential risks and benefits of the treatment before enrolling. Will I get in trouble? Will I be forced to continue participating, even if I'm not comfortable doing so?"

Fact: You can choose to stop participating in a clinical trial and leave at any time.

To answer the above questions: *no*. Put simply, you can choose to stop participating in a clinical trial at any time—even after signing a consent form.

As stated before, voluntarism is one of the core principles of clinical trials. This means that every participant is there of his or her own accord. Clinical trial researchers and coordinators cannot and will never force you to continue participating in a trial if you're no longer comfortable doing so. Regardless of whether you experience adverse side effects, find the treatment more uncomfortable than expected, or are no longer able to attend all of the necessary appointments, you have every right to discontinue the trial. In fact, you can stop participating and leave a clinical trial for any reason and at any time—no questions asked.

The FDA requires that all potential participants be given certain information before enrolling in a clinical trial. Aside from many of the details discussed above, this includes information about the voluntary nature of the trial, including the facts that:

• Research subject participation is voluntary,

- Research subjects have the right to refuse treatment
  and will not lose any benefits to which they are
  entitled, and
- Research subjects may choose to stop participation
  in the clinical trial at any time without losing
  benefits to which they are entitled (such as
  reimbursement or stipends).

You will be made aware of all of this information during the informed consent process. It will be presented to you in the consent document and further explained, if necessary, by the trial's researchers and coordinators. It's important to note that the document will also outline any consequences of leaving a clinical trial before it has been completed, if relevant. That way, you'll know not only that you can quit at any time, but also what the process of quitting might look like if you choose to do so. In some cases, for instance, a trial's procedures may require a slow, organized end of participation. This is often the case if the treatment patients are receiving requires them to taper off (rather than stop the treatment abruptly) in order to prevent symptoms of withdrawal.

Some clinical trials also require that participants sign a new consent form at some point during the study. This can occur when a research team has made a new discovery that might pertain to your health, overall well-being, or any other factor over the course of a trial. As with the initial consent document, it's entirely up to you to decide whether or not you would like to sign a new form. If you decide not to, you are free to discontinue participation in the trial.

To reiterate, you will never be forced to continue participating in a clinical trial that is no longer feasible, regardless of the reason. Even after you sign an initial consent form or an additional consent form during the trial, you have every right to leave at any time.

And as always, I encourage potential and current participants in clinical trials to ask trial researchers and coordinators each and every question they have. No question is too simple, too complex, or too burdensome. Knowledge is power; knowing as much as you can about a study (and asking questions when you are unsure about something) equips you to make the right decision about participating in a clinical trial—or continuing to participate in one.

Myth: "Clinical research teams will pressure me to sign a consent form and enroll in a study, even if I'm not sure about it."

As stated in the previous chapter, researchers and coordinators frequently offer incentives to participants, such as financial compensation and stipends, in order to facilitate participation in clinical trials. With all this encouragement and incentivization, it may appear that clinical research teams are desperate for volunteers and would do just about anything to recruit participants—including pressuring them to enroll in studies.

Fact: No one can force you to participate in a clinical trial.

While research teams are always looking for volunteers, they would never force or coerce anyone into participating in a study. Clinical trials rely entirely on consensual volunteering and participation. This kind of deception would go against everything that clinical trials stand for. It would negate the years and years of work that have gone into ensuring that clinical trials are as transparent and ethical as they are today.

To prevent this from happening, the FDA has established strict guidelines for obtaining informed consent. First and foremost, if you do not sign a consent form voluntarily, then your consent is not considered ethical or valid. The FDA states that a clinical investigator should only obtain consent from a potential participant if they have had enough time to consider whether or not to participate and have not been persuaded or influenced by the investigator. Additionally, researchers must implement special precautions (such as approval by an institutional review board [IRB] or independent ethics committee [IEC]) if they believe that you may have been unfairly influenced by any outside source—including themselves.

Other considerations are taken into account when determining whether your consent was obtained voluntarily, including:[2]

- Illness-related concerns, such as severe mental disorders or the psychological fears that may come with severe or incurable diseases,
- An individual's intellectual and emotional maturity and capability to make complex decisions,
- Religious and cultural values and beliefs,
- A patient's relationship with their caregiver, including financial and care burdens, and
- Undue coercion or influence for research participation.

It's also important that clinical research teams consider the conditions under which a patient provides consent. There may, for example, be a certain degree of pressure involved in being in a clinical setting or laboratory or meeting with groups of people who are eager to find participants for their studies.[3] This is why potential participants are always given the opportunity to take documentation home and/or review it with a third-party expert before signing anything. You're also welcome to bring someone along with you to help you at your appointment, such as a family member, close friend, or caregiver—anyone you trust to help you make important decisions. They will be able to help you keep track of all the information provided to you and help ensure that the final decision you make is yours and no one else's.

Several other considerations must be taken into account to ensure that a person's decision to enroll in a clinical trial is completely voluntary. Minors, for instance, cannot sign informed consent forms for themselves. This is to ensure that external influences (particularly, unfamiliar and potentially intimidating clinical research environments) don't pressure them into doing so.

However, it is important to note that research indicates that most people don't feel external pressure to participate in clinical trials. One study conducted by *Neuro-Oncology*, for instance, found that the vast majority (90%) of patients "didn't feel any pressure from any source to participate or not to participate in [the] clinical trial," while the two patients in the study who did feel pressure said it came from themselves.[4] However, this doesn't mean that ensuring voluntary participation shouldn't be a concern. It's still the responsibility of clinical trial researchers, coordinators, and practice owners like myself to help give patients all the information they need—then let them make the decision to participate on their own.

"CLINICAL TRIALS ARE DANGEROUS."

Many people considering participating in clinical trials worry that the interventions being tested are dangerous or of unknown safety. They (incorrectly) assume that clinical researchers simply don't know how safe an intervention is or whether the intervention being tested is safe for use in humans at all.

It's true that clinical trials are designed for the purpose of researching newly developed treatments. And, as with any medication or treatment, there will be some level of risk involved in receiving them. However, the same is true of any drug you take—even those in your local pharmacy that have already been approved by the FDA.

Let's say that you've been prescribed a topical steroid cream for a skin condition like psoriasis. While helpful in the short term, corticosteroids can be damaging when used for long periods of time. Your dermatologist knows this. He or she will let you know how long to use the cream to obtain the most benefits from it while causing the fewest possible side effects.

Or, perhaps, you take a daily anti-seizure medication. When you first started this drug, you may have experienced unpleasant (but relatively common) side effects, like an upset stomach, dizziness, or even blurred vision. Or, if you're part of an even smaller portion of the population, your anti-seizure drug may have caused an idiosyncratic (unexpected) side effect, such as a skin rash, low white blood cell count, or low platelet count.

Whatever the case may be, you've likely experienced occasional side effects from the medications you've taken in your life. And even if you haven't experienced them firsthand, your doctor —as well as medications' FDA-regulated prescription labels— will have made you aware of the adverse effects medications may have. The fact of the matter is, when taken in certain doses or for certain lengths of time, all medications have the potential to have negative effects on the body.

The same goes for the medications and treatments tested during clinical trials. All medical interventions carry a certain level of risk. But the good news is that you will never go into a clinical trial blind to these risks. Not only have these treatments already been tested for human safety before they've even begun clinical trials, but clinical researchers and coordinators will also have taken care to ensure that you understand each and every potential risk involved with the trial.

Myth: "Clinical trials test medications and treatments that are extremely dangerous or haven't been proven to be safe."

People don't want to gamble with their health. Especially if they're already living with a chronic or debilitating health issue (as are many people interested in clinical trials), the possibility of further impacting their health is a risk that's much too big for many people.

Because of this, many people who express interest in clinical trials have come to me with concerns about the treatments being tested. The prevailing fear I see is that the experimental drugs or treatments undergoing trials are unlikely to be safe, have not been proven to be safe, or are downright dangerous.

Truth be told, this concern can be challenging to address. As I've explained, there is a certain level of risk involved in medical interventions of all kinds. Even FDA-approved over-the-counter and prescription treatments already on the market can have adverse (and sometimes serious) side effects. The interventions going through clinical trials, in particular, have only been tested in a limited capacity; as a result, they carry somewhat of a higher degree of risk than drugs that have been on the market for decades.

Part of the solution to this concern lies in your willingness to work with researchers, coordinators, and your doctor to weigh the pros and cons of participating in a particular clinical trial. You'll need to answer some questions yourself, such as: What are the potential benefits of the treatment being tested? What are the potential risks, and how big of a concern are they to you? In some cases, individuals decide not to participate in clinical trials because they fear a treatment may further impact their health status; in others, they opt out simply because they think the treatment may not offer any worthwhile benefits.

But perhaps the more direct answer to this concern comes from the fact that all new drugs, treatments, and other interventions undergo strict, extensive testing before they're even tested in human trials.

Fact: The interventions tested in clinical trials undergo rigorous screening and testing processes before being administered to patients.

Human testing is just one of the many stages a new treatment goes through before it reaches the market. And because health and safety are of the utmost importance in the medical community, human testing is not the first step in determining an intervention's safety or efficacy. Before a newly developed treatment can be given to clinical trial volunteers, researchers must complete an extensive screening and preclinical testing process. This process alone is so rigorous that it can take years to complete.

The preclinical testing process (which takes place during the clinical research phase) serves the purpose of determining whether an investigational treatment is likely to be effective and safe for use in humans. This phase of research is not done on people. Instead, it is performed on living tissues in a test tube or cell culture (called "in vitro") or on animals ("in vivo"). In some cases, computer models may even be used to test drug interactions (referred to as "in silico").

Preclinical testing evaluates many different features of an investigational treatment. Some stages of the research will assess toxicology (the potential adverse effects of the substance, which helps determine whether the drug is harmful to living tissue), while others will assess things like the unique chemical makeup of a drug.

Just because a treatment is still being tested and has not yet been approved for commercial distribution doesn't mean that it can be given to humans without the necessary precautions. Investigational treatments are still subject to regulations that ensure clinical trial participants' safety throughout all stages of research. It's only after a treatment has passed preclinical research that it can be given to even a small number of human volunteers. And even then, the FDA must give the treatment approval before it can continue onto larger-scale clinical testing in humans.

In short, the treatments tested in clinical trials are only administered to volunteers when scientists have found sufficient evidence that they may prove beneficial without causing undue side effects.

Myth: "I won't be able to judge the risks involved in a clinical trial until I've already started participating."
Many people believe that they simply don't understand science or medicine thoroughly enough to make well-informed decisions about participating in clinical trials. They fear that

their lack of medical knowledge (and lack of knowledge about the clinical trial process, in particular) will put them at risk of entering a trial much more dangerous than they had hoped it to be.

As with other misconceptions surrounding clinical trials, these fears aren't completely unfounded. It is understandable—and very wise, in fact—that people would prefer to know exactly what they're getting into before participating in something that may affect their health.

But it's important to understand that clinical researchers and trial coordinators don't expect you to have a background in medicine. They know that you may not be familiar with some of the aspects of a clinical trial (or even most of them)—and that's okay. Coordinators and researchers take a number of measures to ensure that you have all the information relevant to a clinical trial—and, more importantly, that you understand it—before you decide to enroll.

Fact: Informed consent and clinical trial coordinators provide you with all the information about a clinical trial, including any potential risks, before you agree to participate.

As discussed in the previous chapter, informed consent is much more than just a document—it's an ongoing process and conversation. Its purpose is to continually ensure that you understand all aspects of the trial in which you're participating. However, the informed consent document itself is still a crucial source of information about a clinical trial. This is particularly true when it comes to the risks associated with a trial.

The FDA requires that all potential participants in a clinical trial be given certain information before enrolling. Included in this mandatory information is:

- A description of all the procedures that will be completed during the clinical trial,

- Information about all experimental procedures to be completed during the trial,
- Descriptions of any predictable risks associated with the investigational treatment, and
- Any possible discomforts that could occur as a result of the research, including injections, blood tests, etc. (and the frequency of these procedures).

Some clinical trials may involve more potential discomfort or risks than others. Such trials are said to pose more than "minimal risk." The FDA defines a trial as being of minimal risk when "the probability and magnitude of harm or discomfort anticipated in the research are not greater in and of themselves than those ordinarily encountered in daily life or during the performance of routine physical or psychological examinations or tests."[1] In other words, an investigational treatment poses a minimal risk if it is no more likely to be harmful or uncomfortable than your usual treatments or healthcare visits.

This definition can present somewhat of a gray area—especially when it comes to people with chronic or severe health conditions. After all, what constitutes an "uncomfortable" procedure may be very different for someone who must regularly inject themselves with medication than it is for someone who has only ever suffered from the occasional cold or seasonal allergies.

Ultimately, however, if the FDA determines that a clinical trial involves more than minimal risk, the following information must be included in its informed consent document:

- An explanation as to whether any compensation or medical treatments are available if injury occurs,
- What this compensation or medical treatment consists of, or
- Where more information about compensation or medical treatment may be found.

Some clinical trials may pose particular risks to certain groups of people. In those cases, it is necessary for investigators to outline said risks and to whom they pertain. For example, the FDA requires that informed consent documents include statements informing patients when a treatment or procedure being researched may involve unexpected risks to a participant or their unborn baby if they are or may become pregnant.

An interesting and little-known fact is that informed consent documents don't just address physical risks—they may also explain the financial risks involved with participating in a clinical trial, if there are any. As explained in Chapter 5, it is a common misconception that participating in a clinical trial requires taking on a financial burden. In some cases, however, unexpected changes may occur that could financially affect a trial's volunteers. In these instances, the FDA requires that informed consent documents include:

- Any reasons why a research subject's participation may be ended by the clinical trial investigator (e.g., failing to follow the requirements of the trial)
- Added costs to the research subject that may result from participating in a trial
- The consequence of leaving a trial before it has been completed (e.g., if the research and procedures require a slow and organized end of participation

You don't have to rely on the informed consent document alone to explain the potential risks of participating in a clinical trial. Clinical trial coordinators are there to help you through every step of the process. It's their job to ensure that you feel confident in the fact that you are not taking on any unexpected risks by enrolling in a trial. They will be your first point of contact if you have any questions or concerns about a clinical trial, including any uncertainties or confusion you may have with its informed consent document.

It's not uncommon for people to be overwhelmed with medical forms like informed consent documents. For this reason, having a person that's there to help you make the most well-informed decision possible can make all the difference when it comes to participating in a clinical trial.

Final thoughts on the risks and benefits of clinical trials

There are risks involved with all medical treatments—this is true for those studied in clinical trials as well as those that have been on the shelf at your local pharmacy store for decades.

Keeping you safe when participating in a clinical trial is a top priority for everyone involved—from researchers and clinicians to everyone in between. This is why the goal of clinical research is to minimize the risks and maximize the benefits associated with investigational treatments. Through preclinical testing, we aspire to be confident in a treatment's safety without unduly risking the safety of the participants.

The most important things you, as a volunteer, can do before enrolling in a clinical trial are to do your research, weigh the trial's risks and benefits, and ask questions. If there's something you don't understand or are unsure about, do everything you can to find the answer. I cannot stress enough that the more you know about something—clinical trials, in particular—the more confident you'll be in your decision about it.

"CLINICAL TRIALS AREN'T RIGHT FOR ME."

I've heard it time and time again: "I just don't think that a clinical trial would be right for me." Of course, this statement isn't always exactly the same—it comes in many iterations (each of the myths below, for instance). But the prevailing sentiment is the same: "Clinical trials are only intended for certain people."

It's a common belief that clinical trials are only "right" (or necessary, or beneficial) for people with chronic or debilitating illnesses, such as cancer. This belief likely stems from the misunderstanding that clinical trials only test aggressive, brand-new interventions meant to treat rare or serious diseases. As I hope is evident by now, this is not true. All newly developed treatments, no matter how low risk, must undergo clinical trials before being approved by the FDA for public use. Countless clinical trials are also conducted on treatments that aren't new—they serve the purpose of observing the potential benefits of combining existing treatments or using them in new ways. The misconception that clinical trials are only intended for those who are chronically ill has undoubtedly prevented far too many people from even considering participating. As I'll explore shortly, clinical trials actually need healthy participants.

Others believe that if there were a clinical trial that could help them, their doctor would have told them about it. But the reality is that this isn't necessarily the case. Unless you have a chronic or serious illness and a care team that's continually looking for clinical trials that may benefit you, it's unlikely that your primary care physician will identify each and every relevant volunteer opportunity. Because of this, it is generally up to you to locate the right clinical trial if you're looking for new treatments.

Ultimately, the world of clinical trials is vast. There is bound to be a trial that's right for you—even if you don't think you're unwell enough to need newly developed treatments. Hopefully, gaining a deeper understanding of the wide variety of clinical trials out there will show you that there likely is one that could benefit you, if you're interested.

Myth: "Being in a clinical trial won't help me."

Many people with chronic or severe health conditions feel frustrated by their current care. If you feel as though you've tried every possible treatment option out there, it can start to seem like nothing will ever work or provide relief. Even the promise of accessing state-of-the-art medications and procedures through clinical trials can seem small if you've been let down by ineffective treatments in the past.

But this isn't the only concern for people who feel that clinical trials simply can't help them. Many individuals that aren't affected by severe or long-term health conditions simply don't see the point of participating in a clinical trial. They may wonder what the point is of taking on the potential risks of participating in a trial if the benefits will be slight or nonexistent.

Fact: You can't know whether a clinical trial might benefit you until you learn more about it.

You know how the saying goes: "Don't knock it till you try

it." While this is admittedly too casual of an approach to take in regard to one's health, there is merit to the notion that you can't discount something until you've proven that it's not worth your time.

The same goes for clinical trials. While I'm not suggesting that each and every individual should participate in a trial, I believe that the number of people positively impacted by clinical studies would drastically increase if more individuals were to look into opportunities for participation.

One thing is certain: clinical trials provide people with access to treatments they've likely never tried before. Depending on the trial, you may have the opportunity to receive an investigational medication or procedure not yet available to people outside the study. In this sense, it is absolutely worth your time to do your research about clinical trials. Some may not be worth your time. If, for instance, you found a clinical trial investigating different dosages of a medication that you've already tried, chances are, you wouldn't feel motivated to participate. If, on the other hand, you were to locate a late-stage clinical trial with a newly developed treatment that has shown promising in previous phases, you may be inclined to look into it further.

It's true that you'll need to weigh the pros and cons of participating in a trial before deciding whether or not to enroll. If you find that the potential risks involved in a certain trial are greater than its potential benefits, you may decide that it's not right for you. That's okay—you have every right to forego participating in a trial that you believe is too risky, no matter your reasoning. And, in some cases, the potential benefits of a clinical trial may not be great enough to justify the amount of time or effort you'll need to devote to participating. But here's where the opportunity arises to consider the secondary benefits of clinical trials.

For one, clinical trials help advance medical knowledge and research. They allow scientists to develop new, more effective treatments for all varieties of health conditions. By observing the effects of new treatments or combinations of therapies, clinical trials help advance our understanding of medical conditions and the best ways of treating them. When you partake in a clinical trial, you directly impact that knowledge. In fact, I've seen many people take great pride in the fact that they've played such a substantial role in helping others with the same health concerns simply by participating.

Some people find other meaningful benefits in volunteering for clinical trials. Many appreciate the opportunity to take an active role in their health care and shape their treatment path. This alone can provide individuals with a much-needed sense of agency and self-advocacy in the face of often unpredictable chronic illnesses. Additionally, participating in a clinical trial often involves meeting with your healthcare team more frequently than usual. Because of this, some people find that they improve their communication and transparency with their care teams as they progress through a clinical trial.

Ultimately, the benefits you seek and receive from participating in a clinical trial will be unique to you. If you're unsure whether participation could actually help you, you may want to ask yourself what you're looking to get out of the process. Are you looking for a promising new intervention that could potentially supplement or replace your current treatment? Or are you interested in helping to improve medical knowledge and understanding of a particular disease and its treatment? No matter what your goals are, you'll likely find the right trial if you're willing to put in the research.

Myth: "If there was a clinical trial that could have helped me, my doctor would have told me about it."

People miss countless opportunities for participating in clinical trials because they think that the right trials will just come to them. After all, isn't it your healthcare provider's responsibility to know about current trials that might benefit you? If they haven't mentioned any clinical trials to you, isn't that just because they haven't located any that would be a good fit for your current treatment plan?

Fact: You are your best advocate when it comes to finding clinical trials that could benefit you.

Put simply, your doctor may not be aware of all the available clinical trials out there. In fact, they may not understand the process of selecting and enrolling in clinical trials as well as you will after doing some research.

It's a common misconception that if a clinical trial is being conducted that might be relevant to you, your doctor will bring it to your attention. But it's often the opposite: in many cases, patients find clinical trials that they believe may help them then discuss the possibility of participating with their doctor. While this may seem overwhelming ("How am I to search through the hundreds of thousands of clinical trials that are currently enrolling?"), there are resources available that streamline the trial selection process.

The National Institutes of Health (NIH), for instance, has an online database, ClinicalTrials.gov, that you, your family, or your doctor can use to find appropriate clinical trials. This database lets you search for studies by country, condition or disease, the drug being investigated, and more. The site's advanced search option is even more specific, allowing you to filter clinical trials by things like their eligibility criteria, recruitment status, and phase, making finding the right trial for you even easier. Keep in mind that, as the NIH notes, listing a study on this database does not mean that it has been evaluated by the U.S. Federal Government. For this reason, they advise talking to your healthcare provider and learning about the potential risks and benefits of a specific trial before deciding to enroll.[1]

It's also worth getting in touch with a group like a patient advocacy organization. This type of group can help you navigate the process of finding the right clinical trial. In fact, many of these organizations have tailored services that can assist you in your search and help you discover (and, more importantly, understand) all the options available to you. The Patient Advocate Foundation (Patient-Foundation.org) is a wonderful place to start. They have a wealth of resources available and can help connect you with the right services.

Myth: "Clinical trials are only meant for people who have no other treatment options left."

It makes sense that people often turn to clinical trials when they've exhausted all their standard treatment options. This isn't simply out of desperation or an unwillingness to try alternative methods. Rather, they understand that participating in a clinical trial will give them access to treatments not yet on the market, as well as a high standard of care and monitoring throughout the trial.

But by no means are clinical trials limited to those who feel that they are out of options. In fact, it's often recommended that individuals with chronic illnesses and common ailments alike consider participating in clinical trials early on in their course of treatment.

Fact: Individuals are encouraged to consider participating in clinical trials well before they've exhausted all their treatment options.

It's true that clinical trials often benefit individuals whose standard care (i.e., the treatments normally used for their health condition) hasn't resulted in clinical benefit (improvement to their health). Clinical trials are also beneficial to patients whose conditions do not yet have standard care, as well as those for whom current therapies aren't yielding good results. That said, it's a great idea to explore clinical trial options early on in the course of your disease and treatment—even if other standard therapies are already available to you.

You may, for instance, be eligible for a clinical trial that aims to improve a standard drug or treatment by adding a new agent to it. By participating in such a study, you will continue to receive your current care with the hope that the addition of a new (novel) intervention will result in even greater benefits to your health. In other cases, studies provide patients with the option to receive promising new drugs or treatments during the trial, and then, after the trial has completed, go back to using their standard therapies (which, as we will discuss next, are always available to patients if the interventions being tested aren't successful).

What's more, there are all sorts of clinical trials out there, including those for healthy people and those designed to prevent or diagnose certain medical conditions. Some studies, for instance, aim to establish methods of preventing diseases in people who are at higher risk of developing them, such as genetically linked disorders and hereditary cancers. Other studies focus on developing new techniques for more accurately detecting and diagnosing medical conditions, while others still focus on improving quality of life in people with advanced-stage illnesses or survivors of serious diseases like cancer.

In short, while some clinical trials are reserved for individuals who have exhausted all of the existing treatments for their disease, many studies are open to patients in other situations and at different stages in their healthcare journeys.

Myth: "I'll have to stop using my standard medications and treatments in order to participate in a clinical trial."

A common (and understandable) worry among people considering participating in clinical trials is that they will have to give up their current treatments in order to enroll in a study. While the promise of new, state-of-the-art interventions is often what attracts people to clinical trials, the thought of having to discontinue their medications or therapies—especially if they are finally working well—is enough to dissuade them from participating altogether.

Fact: Many clinical trials allow you to continue with your current treatments while enrolled.

There is a specific type of clinical trial called a nontherapeutic study. People are often unaware of these studies. In fact, many people don't know what they are, as they believe clinical trials serve the sole purpose of testing newly developed medications and treatments. While this is true of therapeutic studies, nontherapeutic clinical trials do not involve administering interventions to patients and testing their effects. Because of this, many nontherapeutic studies can be done while patients continue to receive their standard therapies.

Nontherapeutic studies are conducted with the goal of gathering more information about interventions and health conditions and their impacts on individuals. Some nontherapeutic studies, for instance, may observe the long-term health effects of aggressive medical treatments like chemotherapy, while others may investigate certain aspects of a particular type of tumor. The information gathered from these types of studies is often used to inform the development of new medical interventions. As a result, nontherapeutic trials often lead to therapeutic clinical trials during which these new interventions are tested.

While the majority of nontherapeutic studies allow you to continue with your usual treatments, some clinical trials actually include standard therapies as part of their research. In these studies, participants are able to continue using their existing therapies while being monitored as part of the trial. Furthermore, regardless of the type of study, participants often continue to see their usual care teams while enrolled in clinical trials. Maintaining communication and coordination between an individual's primary healthcare providers and the clinical research team helps ensure that the interventions being studied in a trial will not have any adverse interactions with the patient's standard medications or treatments.

Final thoughts on who can benefit from clinical trials

It's my firm belief that there is a clinical trial out there for everyone that's interested in participating. Of course, I would not attempt to persuade someone truly uncomfortable with volunteering into doing so, regardless of their reasoning. However, I strongly encourage individuals to at least consider the process because there is simply so much to gain from participation.

You don't have to be struggling to find affordable healthcare or dealing with a chronic or debilitating illness to join a clinical trial. Whether you've tried to quit smoking multiple times and just haven't found an approach that's worked, can't seem to get rid of your seasonal allergies, or simply want to help further medical knowledge and bring life-saving treatments to market, the benefits of enrolling in a clinical trial are many.

PART III

LOOKING TO THE FUTURE

CLINICAL TRIALS IN THE AGE OF PANDEMICS

In October of 2019, something peculiar happened during an influenza study at Infinite Clinical Trials. The study's purpose was to test the safety and efficacy of a new flu treatment intended to replace Tamiflu (oseltamivir phosphate). All of the trial's participants were actively experiencing flu-like symptoms (fevers, body aches, cough, fatigue, etc.). Of course, we believed they had the flu.

That said, we still needed to confirm that the participants did, in fact, have influenza. Working with two urgent care centers, we administered rapid flu tests to all patients participating in the trial. As the trial progressed, however, my coworkers and I grew more and more perplexed. This routine flu season trial took a turn for the unexpected—each and every patient tested negative for influenza.

It might seem obvious, in retrospect, that these patients had been infected with SARS-CoV-2 (the virus that causes COVID-19). But at the time, there was no evidence to lead us to believe that a new, rapidly spreading virus was to blame. The novel coronavirus wasn't identified in Wuhan, China, until December of 2019, and the first confirmed case of COVID-19 didn't occur in the United States until a month later, on January 20, 2020. It wasn't until much later that the possibility of my patients having COVID-19 became plausible.

In November of 2020, findings from the U.S. Centers for Disease Control and Prevention (CDC) were published indicating that the virus likely reached American soil prior to the first confirmed case in January.[1] As the report stated, "SARS-CoV-2 infections may have been present in the U.S. in December 2019, earlier than previously recognized."

The CDC conducted serological testing on blood donations from Americans in nine states collected by the American Red Cross between December 13 and January 17. Of the 7,389 donations tested, 106 were found to have evidence of SARS-CoV-2-reactive antibodies. The presence of these antibodies in a person's blood indicates that they have been exposed to COVID-19 because their immune system triggered a defense response against the novel coronavirus. Evidence of SARS-CoV-2-reactive antibodies was detected in 39 blood samples from California, Oregon, and Washington as early as December 13–16 and in 67 samples from Connecticut, Iowa, Massachusetts, Michigan, Rhode Island, and Wisconsin in early January. The latter set of antibodies was found to have been present months before widespread outbreaks occurred in those six states. This means that COVID-19 arrived in the States much earlier than we originally thought—at least several months before its rampant spread led to a nationwide panic, stay-at-home orders, and mask mandates.

Experts aren't sure just how early the novel coronavirus struck North America, nor are they certain exactly how it started. Identifying the origins of a virus (its epidemiology) can be a multi-year endeavor. Epidemiologists have hypothesized that the virus could be traced back to a meat market in Wuhan, China. But as Columbia University virologist Angela Rasmussen admitted, "Finding an animal with a SARS-CoV-2 infection is like looking for a needle in the world's largest haystack. They may never find a 'smoking bat.'"[2]

How clinical trials took the stage in 2020

At this time of writing, COVID-19 has claimed the lives of well over 500,000 Americans and more than 3 million souls worldwide. It has wreaked havoc on global economies, uprooted our daily lives, and isolated us from the ones we love most. It has touched all of our lives and communities. But what we have ultimately learned during this time is that we must come together in spirit in order to rise above this crisis as one.

In a true testament to the innate resilience and proactivity of humanity, it didn't take long for researchers, institutions, private companies, and grantors to unite in the battle against COVID-19. Early on in the pandemic, researchers designed an astounding 1,200 clinical studies to test preventive measures and treatments for the novel coronavirus. While many were small and uncontrolled (making them unlikely to yield reliable results and insights),[3] the studies nonetheless led to some extraordinary breakthroughs.

Not even a month after the first identified COVID-19 cases, a Chinese research team succeeded in sequencing the novel coronavirus, sharing their findings with the World Health Organization (WHO) between January 11–12.[4] Since then, an unprecedented level of collaboration and coordination encouraged researchers worldwide to share their data in open-access journals. Of course, they also continued to rely on clinical trials for breakthroughs. One type of clinical trial, in particular, helped us make faster, more reliable advancements in COVID-19 research: the *adaptive platform trial.*

Adaptive platform trials allow researchers to test multiple experimental interventions at the same time against a single shared control group. And, as the name of this type of study suggests, it is highly adaptable and adjustable. More specifically, the FDA defines an "adaptive design" as "a clinical trial design that allows for prospectively planned modifications to one or more aspects of the design based on accumulating data from subjects in the trial."[5] In other words, an adaptive clinical trial is one that has been designed to allow for as-needed changes—researchers, for example, can add or remove interventions and even alter the design of an adaptive platform trial as new discoveries are made.

As you can surely imagine, the flexibility of adaptive trials has proven invaluable in a situation as rapidly evolving and unpredictable as the COVID-19 pandemic. Such clinical trials were responsible for many of the breakthroughs in practical treatment and disease prevention achieved in 2020. In April, for example, the National Institutes of Health's Adaptive COVID-19 Treatment Trial (ACTT) demonstrated the efficacy of an antiviral agent, Remdesivir, in speeding up recovery time and even potentially reducing mortality.[6] Just weeks later, in June, another adaptive trial in the U.K. called RECOVERY (Randomised Evaluation of COVid-19 thERapY) found that the common steroid Dexamethasone reduced mortality among patients hospitalized with COVID-19.[7] It also showed that other treatments, including a combination of the HIV treatments Lopinavir and Ritonavir, were ineffective in treating the virus. Aside from their practical applications, these findings were valuable for the simple fact that they provided clarity and hope in a time of widespread uncertainty and fear.

Each and every achievement made during these months of research was vital. They were the direct result of the collaboration and dedication of scientists, research coordinators, grantors, and, of course, *clinical trial volunteers*. These achievements wouldn't have been possible without them.

Yet, despite these optimistic breakthroughs, a worrying trend has arisen since the beginning of 2020. As greater numbers of COVID-19 trials began to make front-page headlines, clinical trials found their way into the broader American consciousness. Especially as vaccine trials become part of everyday conversation, clinical trials began to dominate public discourse in a way that industry professionals have never experienced. This newfound interest in clinical trials is very welcome. Unfortunately, it has also come with a healthy dose of skepticism.

Just as quickly as they were praised for advancing the fight against COVID-19, clinical trials began to come under fire. They became politicized and stigmatized. I experienced this first-hand when I received backlash for the interviews I gave encouraging Black Americans to participate in COVID-19 trials. Several times in 2020, I was asked at the eleventh hour not to attend COVID testing events for fear that my practice's presence alone would spark controversy or make attendees uncomfortable. It's hard to put into words how much this has pained me. I never thought I would witness this much fear, anger, or distrust surrounding clinical trials.

This response is one of the biggest factors behind my decision to write this book. During the pandemic, clinical trials became more important than ever. And, as we will now explore, this is especially true for Black Americans.

Why Black Americans' participation in clinical trials is so crucial

I know fully well that encouraging more Black Americans to participate in clinical trials will not be an easy task. I believe, however, that the COVID-19 pandemic presented us with the best possible evidence that our involvement in the clinical trial process is absolutely vital.

Mounting evidence has shown that certain racial and ethnic minority populations have been disproportionately affected by COVID-19. The CDC identified the multitude of long-standing, systemic social and health inequities that contributed to an increased risk of contracting and dying from COVID-19 for minority groups, including:[8]

- **Lack of access to and underutilization of healthcare services:** A number of factors can limit

minority populations' access to comprehensive
healthcare, including communication and language
barriers, cultural differences between patients and
healthcare providers, lack of transportation or the
ability to take time off from work, and historical,
ongoing discrimination and inequity within the
healthcare industry.

What's more, people from certain racial and ethnic minority
populations are more likely to be uninsured than non-Hispanic
Whites. They may also hesitate to seek healthcare services. This
can, in many cases, be attributed to a lack of trust in the government and healthcare systems responsible for their inequitable
treatment. This hesitation also finds its roots in historical atroci-
ties, including the Tuskegee experiments and forced sterilization
of minority populations.[9]

- **Discrimination:** While strides have been made in
  the ongoing fight for equity, systemic
  discrimination still persists in many sectors, such as
  healthcare, housing, and finance. Overt
  discrimination (i.e., racist actions) and systemic
  inequalities lead to chronic stress and anxiety. They
  also impact social and economic factors that
  increase the risk of COVID-19 spread among
  minority populations.
- **Educational, income, and wealth gaps and
  disparities:** A lack of access to quality education can
  lead to lower high school completion rates and
  barriers to entering higher education in minority
  populations. This can limit future career
  opportunities, forcing individuals to accept lower-
  paying and/or less stable jobs. People with limited
  job opportunities are less likely to leave their jobs,
  which may put them at higher risk of exposure to

SARS-CoV-2 because they cannot afford to miss work, even if they're ill.

- **Occupation:** Minority populations are disproportionately represented in essential and blue-collar occupations, such as in public transportation, healthcare, and grocery stores. These types of jobs can put people at higher risk of exposure to viruses like SARS-CoV-2 for any number of reasons. They may require employees to be in close proximity to colleagues and customers and often do not provide the option of working from home.

- **Housing:** Individuals in minority groups may have no choice but to live in crowded conditions, making it difficult to follow social distancing rules and other COVID-19 prevention protocols. Additionally, disproportionate and increasing unemployment rates among certain racial and ethnic groups during the COVID-19 pandemic may have contributed to a greater risk of eviction, leading to homelessness or cohabitation (shared housing).

The degree to which COVID-19 has disproportionately impacted people of color is astounding. In an eye-opening ongoing report titled "The Color of Coronavirus," the APM Research Lab continues to analyze COVID-19 deaths in the U.S. by race and ethnicity. Having documented the race and ethnicity of 94% of the cumulative deaths from COVID-19 in the United States, the Lab's latest update reveals that Black, Pacific Islander, and Indigenous Americans have suffered the greatest loss of life.[10]

Ultimately, Black, Pacific Islander, Indigenous, and Latino/a Americans have experienced double or more the COVID-19 death rate of White Americans, who experience the lowest age-adjusted death rates. In just four weeks from late October to mid-November 2020, for example, 1 in 875 Black Americans died (114.3 deaths per 100,000 people), compared to 1 in 1,625 White Americans (61.7 deaths per 100,000 people). If these minority groups had the same COVID-19 mortality rates as White Americans, about 21,200 Black, 10,000 Latino/a, 1,000 Indigenous, and 70 Pacific Islander Americans would still be alive.

Despite these deeply upsetting facts, a lack of diversity in clinical trials for COVID-19 remained a problem throughout the pandemic. Black Americans, in particular, were underrepresented in these trials. This was the case for both interventional studies and observational studies (which analyze patient outcomes in relation to treatments currently being used for COVID-19). In the pharmaceutical company Pfizer's COVID-19 vaccine trials, for instance, just 8% of participants were Black.[11] Although Black Americans account for more than 13% of the U.S. population, they make up a much smaller percentage of clinical trial participants.

Black Americans, in particular, have slower metabolic rates than White Americans.[12,13] The fact that we metabolize drugs differently than others impacts the way in which these drugs affect us. If very few Black Americans participate in clinical trials, we cannot be sure of the efficacy of new treatments or vaccines in our populations, even if they do reach the market.

I'm using COVID-19 here as a case study. But the truth is that diverse representation in clinical trials will always be an essential part of the process for developing the best possible medications and treatments. If we are to find a successful treatment or vaccine for COVID-19, we need to be sure that it will work for everyone—not just select populations—because people of different races and ethnicities respond differently to certain treatments.

CLINICAL TRIALS TODAY, TOMORROW, AND BEYOND

As one of the few African American women in the clinical trials space, I've taken it upon myself as a personal responsibility, of sorts, to do what I can to help bring a better understanding of clinical trials to people of color.

Infinite Clinical Trials is considered a "high enrollment site." My staff is extremely dedicated to (and good at) what they do. And while my team puts their great effort into recruiting volunteers, I've also spent many of my own hours sharing information about clinical trials in the hopes of bringing the opportunity to participate to those who need it most.

We also rely heavily on social media to spread the word about currently enrolling clinical trials. In fact, this is one of the biggest ways in which potential patients find us. And we don't just use social media to recruit participants—we also distribute a great deal of educational information. *What are clinical trials? Why are they important?* These are the two most commonly asked questions at my practice and many others, and just two of the myriad questions we answer through a variety of widely accessible content we publish and share.

The biggest focus in our educational content and social media efforts is to highlight minority participation in clinical trials. We want to build confidence, trust, and understanding around what we're offering. As explored earlier, Americans of color—and, in particular, Black Americans—have every right to be wary of the healthcare and clinical trials industries. It's understandable that many minorities choose not to put themselves and their health on the line (as they understand to be the case when, say, volunteering for a clinical trial) after repeated and systemic abuse and deception. I feel that it's my job, as someone on the "inside" of both clinical trials and the minority population, to help rebuild this broken trust (if there even was a sufficient degree of trust, to begin with).

At the end of the day, we need more minority participation in clinical trials. This is true of all clinical trials, but—as I hope I've shown—it was more important for COVID-19 trials than any other.

I personally know many people who have been affected by COVID-19. I have, as of now, lost seven family members to the virus. Several more have faced serious health complications from the disease. And much to my dismay (and that of others in the medical field), I simply cannot predict how anyone will respond to it. I've seen entirely healthy family members of middle age require weeks of ventilation, while others of an older age with underlying health conditions have had only minimal symptoms.

I should note here that I don't write this for sympathy. I am sharing this to preface the fact that, for those readers who haven't lost anyone to COVID-19 or known anyone affected by it, the hardest part is not knowing how someone will respond to the virus once they've been infected with it. We just can't predict who will recover from the disease and who will not. It's a disheartening and troubling fact.

Evidently, there is much more to be learned about this disease before we can fully understand its effects on different individuals. And this is, in part, why I hold so much hope that more people will become involved in clinical trials. The only way we can gain the knowledge needed to fully eradicate diseases like this is to study the effects of treatments and vaccines on humans.

And yet, despite the most devastating effects of COVID-19 and the most promising clinical trials, many Americans remain wary about deciding to receive a vaccine. The prevailing sentiment among many skeptics is that the vaccines being offered were developed much too quickly to be safe or trustworthy. Of course, as I've addressed, the factors contributing to distrust of the healthcare system are many and complex. And distrust of pharmaceutical companies—which are, inherently, profiting from the interventions they develop—is another (not entirely separate) issue. But to those questioning whether we had "enough time" to develop vaccines that are not only effective in preventing COVID-19, but also safe for humans, I'll say this: firstly, it wasn't actually as quick as many people think.

While quarantine and nationwide shutdowns somewhat skewed our perception of time, it's been more than a year since scientists first started developing vaccines for SARS-CoV-2. Each vaccine on the market has gone through the same channels and phases as every flu, measles, and smallpox vaccine you've received. The only reason that developing COVID-19 was expedited was that doing so took absolute precedence over countless other projects in the medical community. So many other treatments being tested were paused to devote resources to finding a vaccine for this virus. Almost immediately after global concerns about the novel coronavirus arose, members of the scientific community began committing all of their hours to developing a vaccine. It became an "all-hands-on-deck" situation, with researchers working around the clock for many more hours than they would in a "normal" week. We have taken all the same precautions, jumped through all the same hoops, and conducted all the same testing necessary to prove that these vaccines are both effective and safe. The process has just been expedited due to the sheer gravity of the pandemic.

And to those doubting the integrity of the pharmaceutical

industry and the companies backing the development of these vaccines, I'll posit this: those that have released vaccines are reputable, world-renowned companies that have worked for decades and decades to build their brands. What motive would they have for putting something on the market that's not only unsafe but also intentionally designed to hurt someone? Companies like Moderna, Pfizer, and Johnson & Johnson already have hundreds of thousands of medications and interventions on the market. They have no reason to put their reputations in the medical community on the line—especially when it comes to something as momentous as this.

Ultimately, my goal—and the goal of so many others in the healthcare field—is to help, not to hurt. To encourage and educate, not force or persuade. The decision to participate in a clinical trial is yours; I only hope to provide you with the information needed to make the most well-informed decision possible.

ACKNOWLEDGMENTS

This book was written thanks to the combined effort, support, and love of many people in my life. I would like to thank just a few of them individually.

To my grandmother: You have always encouraged me to go after my dreams, even when others have questioned my path. You supported me, prayed for me, and uplifted me every day of your life; for that, I will always be grateful.

To my mother: You are my rock—my unending source of support. I thank you, love you, and appreciate you for every sacrifice and prayer. You have allowed me to run my business while navigating single motherhood. Without you, I would not be where I am today. You inspire me to reach for my dreams and to aim for the stars.

To my three beautiful daughters, Sorea, Calia, and Wynter: You are the lights of my life. You keep me going, and I cannot wait to see the young women you will become. I want you to understand the time, effort, and dedication it takes to make yourself and this world a better place. Strive to grow and help others in everything that you do—that will make me so proud of you.

To my staff: Infinite Clinical Trials would not exist without your dedication, hard work, and care. Thank you for all that you do each and every day. You have given me the opportunity to lead a group of wonderful individuals—to be a leader of great leaders.

To Victoria: I would like to express my special thanks and gratitude. You saw my vision and helped me bring this book to life. You helped me in gathering information, collecting data, and editing my work. Despite your busy schedule, you provided many ideas in making this project unique. Your feedback and support have been invaluable. It was a labor of love, and we saw each other through it.

To everyone who reads this book and shares it with others: I give you the deepest, sincerest thanks. I appreciate you.

Lastly, I give God all the glory for my experiences, my courage, and my knowledge. Thank you, God, for instilling in me the gift of genuine care to help bring new medications and medical devices to those who need them.

ABOUT THE AUTHOR

Calethia T. Hodges is the founder and CEO of Infinite Clinical Trials, LLC, two clinical research firms outside Atlanta, GA. In addition to running two research sites, Hodges also prepares future clinical research professionals for employment opportunities through the company's externship program and partner universities, which place graduates with other leading CROs in the pharmaceutical and biologics industry.

One of the few African American women in her field, Ms. Hodges obtained her Bachelor of Science at DePaul University and holds professional certificates in Clinical Trials Monitoring, Obtaining Approval for Clinical Trials in the United States and European Union, and Clinical Trials Management. She is an active member of the Association of Clinical Research Professionals (ACRP), Society of Clinical Research Associates (SOCRA), and Society for Clinical Research Sites (SCRC).

Hodges and her three daughters live near Atlanta. She enjoys traveling, swimming, reading, and writing. Her daughters are very active in sports, which keeps her days busy and filled with joy.

NOTES

Author's Note

1. *U.S. Census Bureau QuickFacts: Atlanta city, Georgia.* (2019). Census Bureau QuickFacts. https://www.census.gov/quickfacts/atlantacitygeorgia
2. Bunn, C. (2020, July 21). A COVID-19 vaccine will work only if trials include Black participants, experts say. NBC News. https://www.nbcnews.com/news/nbcblk/covid-19-vaccine-will-only-work-if-trials-include-black-n1228371
3. Centers for Disease Control and Prevention. (2020, March 2). *Tuskegee Study and Health Benefit Program - CDC - NCHHSTP.* CDC.gov. https://www.cdc.gov/tuskegee/index.html

What Are Clinical Trials?

1. U.S. National Library of Medicine. (2000). *Glossary: Phases of Clinical Trials.* ClinicalTrials.Gov. https://www.clinicaltrials.gov/ct2/help/glossary/phase
2. U.S. National Library of Medicine. *Learn About Clinical Studies.* ClinicalTrials.gov. https://clinicaltrials.gov/ct2/about-studies/learn
3. U.S. Food & Drug Administration. *Informed Consent for Clinical Trials.* FDA.gov. https://www.fda.gov/patients/clinical-trials-what-patients-need-know/informed-consent-clinical-trials
4. U.S. Food & Drug Administration. (2000). *Good Clinical Practice 101: An Introduction* [Slides]. F. https://www.fda.gov/media/77415/download
5. Smith-Tyler, J. (2007). *Informed Consent, Confidentiality, and Subject Rights in Clinical Trials.* Proceedings of the American Thoracic Society, 4(2), 189–193. https://www.atsjournals.org/doi/full/10.1513/pats.200701-008GC
6. U.S. Department of Health and Human Services. (2015, December 18). *What is the difference between "consent" and "authorization" under the HIPAA Privacy Rule?* HHS.Gov. https://www.hhs.gov/hipaa/for-professionals/faq/264/what-is-the-difference-between-consent-and-authorization/index.html

The History of Clinical Trials

1. Collier, R. (2009). Legumes, lemons and streptomycin: A short history of the clinical trial. *Canadian Medical Association Journal,* 180(1), 23–24. https://doi.org/10.1503/cmaj.081879

2. Bull John P. (1951). *A Study of the History and Principles of Clinical Thera-peutic Trials* [MD thesis]. University of Cambridge; 1951. 80 p. https://www.jameslindlibrary.org/wp-data/uploads/2014/05/bull-19511.pdf

3. Gauch, R. R. (2009) "The Clinical Trial –The Gold Standard." In: *It's Great! Oops, No It Isn't*. https://doi.org/10.1007/978-1-4020-8907-7_4

4. Meinert, C. L. (1986). *Clinical Trials: Design, Conduct, and Analysis* (1st ed.). Oxford University Press.

5. Encyclopædia Britannica. (2020). *Lady Mary Wortley Montagu | British author*. Britannica.Com. https://www.britannica.com/biography/Lady-Mary-Wortley-Montagu

6. Riedel, S. (2005). Edward Jenner and the History of Smallpox and Vaccina-tion. *Baylor University Medical Center Proceedings*, 18(1), 21–25. https://doi.org/10.1080/08998280.2005.11928028

7. Dunn, P. M. (1997). James Lind (1716-94) of Edinburgh and the treatment of scurvy. *Archives of Disease in Childhood - Fetal and Neonatal Edition*, 76(1), F64–F65. https://doi.org/10.1136/fn.76.1.f64

8. Brown, S. R. (2003). *Scurvy: How a Surgeon, a Mariner and a Gentleman Solved the Greatest Medical Mystery of the Age of Sail* (First Thus ed.). Summersdale Pub Ltd.

9. The James Lind Library. (2019, May 7). *Lind J (1753)*. https://www.james-lindlibrary.org/lind-j-1753/

10. Rogers, Everett M. (1995). *Diffusion of Innovations* (4th ed.). New York, NY: Free Press.

11. Junod, Ph.D., S. W. *FDA and Clinical Drug Trials: A Short History*. U.S. Food & Drug Administration. https://www.fda.gov/media/110437/download

12. O'Rourke, M. F. (1992). Frederick Akbar Mahomed. *Hypertension*, 19(2), 212–217. https://doi.org/10.1161/01.hyp.19.2.212

13. Crofton, J. (2006). The MRC randomized trial of streptomycin and its legacy: a view from the clinical front line. *Journal of the Royal Society of Medi-cine*, 99(10), 531–534. https://doi.org/10.1258/jrsm.99.10.531

14. World Health Organization. (2018, October 31). *Tuberculosis (TB)*. https://www.who.int/gho/tb/en/

15. Metcalfe, N. H. (2011). Sir Geoffrey Marshall (1887–1982): respiratory physician, catalyst for anaesthesia development, doctor to both Prime Minister and King, and World War I Barge Commander. *Journal of Medical Biography*, 19(1), 10–14. https://doi.org/10.1258/jmb.2010.010019

16. ProPublica. (2020, March 2). *Black Patients Miss Out On Promising Cancer Drugs*. https://www.propublica.org/article/black-patients-miss-out-on-promising-cancer-drugs

17. Shen, M. J., Peterson, E. B., & Costas-Muñiz, R., *et al.* (2017). The Effects of Race and Racial Concordance on Patient-Physician Communication: A Systematic Review of the Literature. *Journal of Racial and Ethnic Health Disparities*, 5(1), 117–140. https://doi.org/10.1007/s40615-017-0350-4

18. Smedley, B. D., Stith, A. Y., Institute of Medicine, Colburn, L., Association of American Medical Colleges, Evans, C. H., & Association of Academic Health Centers. (2001). Increasing Racial and Ethnic Diversity Among Physicians: An Intervention to Address Health Disparities? In *The Right Thing*

to Do, *The Smart Thing to Do: Enhancing Diversity in the Health Professions* (1st ed.). National Academies Press.

19. Lackland, D. T. (2014). Racial Differences in Hypertension: Implications for High Blood Pressure Management. *The American Journal of the Medical Sciences*, 348(2), 135–138. https://doi.org/10.1097/maj.0000000000000308

20. *Tuskegee Study - Research Implications - CDC - NCHHSTP.* (2020, March 2). Centers for Disease Control and Prevention. https://www.cdc.gov/tuskegee/after.htm

Why Are Clinical Trials Important?

1. Wise, J. (2020). Covid-19: Study reveals six clusters of symptoms that could be used as a clinical prediction tool. *BMJ*, m2911. https://doi.org/10.1136/bmj.m2911

2. *HPV-Associated Cancer Statistics.* (2020, September 3). Centers for Disease Control and Prevention. https://www.cdc.gov/cancer/hpv/statistics/index.htm

3. *Human Papillomavirus Vaccine (HPV).* (n.d.). American Academy of Family Physicians. https://www.aafp.org/family-physician/patient-care/prevention-wellness/immunizations-vaccines/disease-pop-immunization/human-papillo-mavirus-vaccine-hpv.html

4. Galimberti, V., Cole, B. F., & Viale, G., *et al.* (2018). Axillary dissection versus no axillary dissection in patients with breast cancer and sentinel-node micrometastases (IBCSG 23-01): 10-year follow-up of a randomised, controlled phase 3 trial. *The Lancet Oncology*, 19(10), 1385–1393. https://doi.org/10.1016/s1470-2045(18)30380-2

The Truth About Clinical Trials

1. Kiesel, L. (2017, October 7). *Women and pain: Disparities in experience and treatment.* Harvard Health Blog. https://www.health.harvard.edu/blog/women-and-pain-disparities-in-experience-and-treatment-2017100912562

2. Scharff, D. P., Mathews, K. J., Jackson, P., Hoffsuemmer, J., Martin, E., & Edwards, D. (2010). More than Tuskegee: Understanding Mistrust about Research Participation. *Journal of Health Care for the Poor and Underserved*, 21(3), 879–897. https://doi.org/10.1353/hpu.0.0323

"Clinical Trial Volunteers Are Mistreated."

1. Institute of Medicine (US) Committee on Health Research and the Privacy of Health Information: The HIPAA Privacy Rule; Nass SJ, Levit LA, Gostin LO, editors. *Beyond the HIPAA Privacy Rule: Enhancing Privacy, Improving Health Through Research.* Washington (DC): National Academies Press (US);

2009. 2, The Value and Importance of Health Information Privacy. Available from: https://www.ncbi.nlm.nih.gov/books/NBK9579/

2. Westin, A. F. & Harris Interactive. (2008, March). *How the Public Views Privacy and Health Research.* https://www.ftc.gov/sites/default/files/documents/public_comments/health-care-delivery-534908-00001/534908-00001.pdf

3. Woolley M, Propst SM. Public attitudes and perceptions about health related research. *JAMA.* 2005;294:1380–1384.

4. Tucker, K., Branson, J., Dilleen, M. *et al.* (2016). Protecting patient privacy when sharing patient-level data from clinical trials. *BMC Med Res Methodol,* 16(S1). https://doi.org/10.1186/s12874-016-0169-4

5. U.S. Department of Health and Human Services. (2013, July 26). Summary of the HIPAA Privacy Rule. HHS.Gov. https://www.hhs.gov/hipaa/for-professionals/privacy/laws-regulations/index.html

"Participating in Clinical Trials Is Expensive."

1. Sertkaya, A., Wong, H.-H., Jessup, A., & Beleche, T. (2016). Key cost drivers of pharmaceutical clinical trials in the United States. *Clinical Trials,* 13(2), 117–126. https://doi.org/10.1177/1740774515625964

2. NIH National Cancer Institute. (2020, February 6). *Insurance Coverage and Clinical Trials.* https://www.cancer.gov/about-cancer/treatment/clinical-trials/paying/insurance

Myths About Informed Consent

1. Davis, T. C., Berkel, H. J., Holcombe, R. F., Pramanik, S., & Divers, S. G. (1998). Informed Consent for Clinical Trials: a Comparative Study of Standard Versus Simplified Forms. *JNCI Journal of the National Cancer Institute,* 90(9), 668–674. https://doi.org/10.1093/jnci/90.9.668

2. Gupta, U. C. (2013). Informed consent in clinical research: Revisiting few concepts and areas. *Perspectives in Clinical Research,* 4(1), 26. https://doi.org/10.4103/2229-3485.106373

3. Roberts, L. W. (2002). Informed Consent and the Capacity for Voluntarism. *American Journal of Psychiatry,* 159(5), 705–712. https://doi.org/10.1176/appi.ajp.159.5.705

4. Knifed, E., Lipsman, N., Mason, W., & Bernstein, M. (2008). Patients' perception of the informed consent process for neurooncology clinical trials. *Neuro-Oncology,* 10(3), 348–354. https://doi.org/10.1215/15228517-2008-007

"Clinical Trials Are Dangerous."

1. Minimal Risk. (2014, August 6). U.S. Food and Drug Administration. https://www.fda.gov/patients/informed-consent-clinical-trials/minimal-risk

"Clinical Trials Aren't Right for Me."

1. *Finding a Clinical Trial.* (2018, November 6). National Institutes of Health (NIH). https://www.nih.gov/health-information/nih-clinical-research-trials-you/finding-clinical-trial

Clinical Trials in the Age of Pandemics

1. Basavaraju, S. V., Patton, M. E., Grimm, K., *et al.* (2020). Serologic testing of U.S. blood donations to identify SARS-CoV-2-reactive antibodies: December 2019-January 2020. *Clinical Infectious Diseases*, ciaa1785, 1–21. https://doi.org/10.1093/cid/ciaa1785
2. Mallapaty, S. (2020). Where did COVID come from? WHO investigation begins but faces challenges. *Nature*, 587(7834), 341–342. https://doi.org/10.1038/d41586-020-03165-9
3. Riglin, E., & Garde, D. (2020, July 6). *Data show panic, disorganization dominate the study of Covid-19 drugs.* STAT. https://www.statnews.com/2020/07/06/data-show-panic-and-disorganization-dominate-the-study-of-covid-19-drugs/
4. World Health Organization. (2020, January 13). *Novel Coronavirus – China.* https://www.who.int/csr/don/12-january-2020-novel-coronavirus-china/en/
5. U.S. Department of Health and Human Services, U.S. Food and Drug Administration, Center for Drug Evaluation and Research (CDER), & Center for Biologics Evaluation and Research (CBER). (2019, November). *Adaptive Designs for Clinical Trials of Drugs and Biologics: Guidance for Industry.* https://www.fda.gov/regulatory-information/search-fda-guidance-documents/adaptive-design-clinical-trials-drugs-and-biologics-guidance-industry
6. National Institutes of Health. (2020, April 29). *NIH clinical trial shows Remdesivir accelerates recovery from advanced COVID-19.* National Institutes of Health (NIH). https://www.nih.gov/news-events/news-releases/nih-clinical-trial-shows-remdesivir-accelerates-recovery-advanced-covid-19
7. University of Oxford. (2020, June 16). *Low-cost dexamethasone reduces death by up to one third in hospitalised patients with severe respiratory complications of COVID-19.* RECOVERY: Randomised Evaluation of COVID-19 Therapy. https://www.recoverytrial.net/news/low-cost-dexamethasone-reduces-death-by-up-to-one-third-in-hospitalised-patients-with-severe-respiratory-complications-of-covid-19

8. Centers for Disease Control and Prevention. (2020, July 24). *Health Equity Considerations and Racial and Ethnic Minority Groups.* https://www.cdc.gov/coronavirus/2019-ncov/community/health-equity/race-ethnicity.html

9. Stern, A. M. (2005). STERILIZED in the Name of Public Health: Race, Immigration, and Reproductive Control in Modern California. *American Journal of Public Health,* 95(7), 1128–1138. https://doi.org/10.2105/AJPH.2004.041608

10. APM Research Lab. (2020, November). *The Color of Coronavirus: COVID-19 Deaths by Race and Ethnicity in the United States.* https://www.apmresearchlab.org/covid/deaths-by-race

11. Borno, H. T., Zhang, S., & Gomez, S. (2020). COVID-19 disparities: An urgent call for race reporting and representation in clinical research. *Contemporary Clinical Trials Communications,* 19, 100630. https://doi.org/10.1016/j.conctc.2020.100630

12. Sharp, T. A., Bell, M. L., & Grunwald, G. K., *et al.*. (2002). Differences in Resting Metabolic Rate between White and African-American Young Adults. *Obesity Research,* 10(8), 726–732. https://doi.org/10.1038/oby.2002.99

13. Weyer, C., Snitker, S., Bogardus, C., & Ravussin, E. (1999). Energy metabolism in African Americans: potential risk factors for obesity. *The American Journal of Clinical Nutrition,* 70(1), 13–20. https://doi.org/10.1093/ajcn/70.1.13